D0400901

"I Flunked My Mammogram!"

What you need to know about breast cancer

NOW!

"I Flunked My Mammogram!"

What you need to know about breast cancer

NOW!

Ernie Bodai, M.D. F.A.C.S.
with
Richard A. Zmuda

B2Z Publishing, Inc.
Severna Park, Maryland

Copyright © 2001 Ernie Bodai, MD and Richard A. Zmuda

All rights reserved. No part of this book shall be reproduced, stored in a retrieval system or transmitted by any means, electronic, mechanical, photocopying, recording or otherwise, without written permission from the publisher.

"I Flunked My Mammogram!" is a registered trademark of B2Z Publishing.

International Standard Book Number (ISBN): 0-9712070-0-3
Library of Congress Catalog Card Number: Available upon request.
Printed in the United States of America.

Note: The information contained herein is for educational purposes only and is intended to provide helpful information to people facing breast cancer risk or undergoing treatment for the disease. The authors have used extensive efforts to ensure that the information is accurate and current. However, advances in medical research and treatment may invalidate certain information. Any person who has or might have a health problem should consult a professional healthcare provider.

B2Z Publishing, Inc.
Post Office Box 307
Severna Park, Maryland 21146 USA
Tel: 1-888-371-1800 (toll free) / 410-431-8894
Web site: www.B2Zpublishing.com
E-mail: towardcure@aol.com

> **A portion of the proceeds from each book will be donated by the authors to support breast cancer education programs.**

The cover depicts a broken DNA strand and the revolutionary efforts by individual researchers to repair it. Also shown is the Breast Cancer Research Stamp, founded by Dr. Ernie Bodai, which has raised over $25 million for breast cancer research. The stamps are available for purchase at all U.S. Post Offices and on the Internet at Stampsonline.com and curebreastcancer.org.

Stamp design © 1998 U.S. Postal Service.
Reproduced with permission. All rights reserved.

Cover design and illustrations by Joshua D. Williams.

Dedication

To the cancer angels who
watch over us all ...

You know who you are.

Forward

By Nancy Brinker
Founding Chair, The Susan G. Komen Breast Cancer Foundation

Frustrated after performing thousands of surgeries on women with breast cancer, Dr. Ernie Bodai, a Sacramento breast cancer surgeon, became determined to personally find a way to quicken the pace of breast cancer research.

During a routine trip to the post office, he came upon a remarkable idea. Noticing a display of commemorative stamps, he wondered if people would be willing to pay a bit extra for a special breast cancer stamp if the surplus would be directed to breast cancer research.

So began a remarkable one-man mission to convince the United States Postal Service (USPS) to issue the first-ever "semi-postal" stamp in the agency's nearly 250-year history. But, as it turns out, the USPS wasn't the most difficult hurdle; approval from the United States Congress was much more challenging.

Undaunted, Dr. Bodai began an exhaustive personal lobbying effort to convince Congress to authorize a special "Breast Cancer Research Stamp" priced at 40 cents—7 cents more than the 33-cent face value at the time. The surplus would be directed toward the National Cancer Institute and the Department of Defense Breast Cancer Research Program.

To the amazement of almost everyone, with the notable exception of Dr. Bodai, Congress passed the "Breast Cancer Research Stamp Act" in July 1997, with the President signing the Act into law only weeks later.

As of this writing, the Breast Cancer Research Stamp has raised over $25 million to fund critical research initiatives. Importantly, the stamp has received a two-year re-authorization through 2002—thanks once again to Dr. Bodai's intensive lobbying efforts and the support of breast cancer advocacy groups such as the Susan G. Komen Breast Cancer Foundation.

In March 2001, the Komen Foundation was proud to honor Dr. Bodai with our prestigious Founder's Award. During the presentation, I praised Dr. Bodai for his extraordinary vision and noted that his efforts "epitomize the public-private partnerships that are necessary for achieving our goal of eradicating breast cancer as a life-threatening disease."

"I Flunked My Mammogram!" is further evidence of Dr. Bodai's invaluable—and indefatigable—efforts on behalf of the hundreds of thousands of women and men who have to confront breast cancer in their daily lives. From the very first pages, readers feel as if they are sitting in Dr. Bodai's office while he calmly explains all of the issues they must now address. *"I Flunked My Mammogram!"* is easy to read and reduces the complexities of this terrible disease to understandable terms. The book answers all the questions so often asked. It will ease your concerns and "hold your hand" as you walk through the chapters.

"I Flunked My Mammogram!" serves both as a wonderful primer for the newly diagnosed patient and her family as well as a continuing resource for the growing number of long-term breast cancer survivors. Read it and you will understand that there is real hope, the hope for a cure.

Nancy Brinker

Acknowledgments

Without question, this book would not have been possible without the extraordinary support of so many wonderful individuals. While this list is certainly not all-inclusive, we feel privileged to have been able to work with the following special people in the publication of *"I Flunked My Mammogram!"*:

Phyllis Avedon	Jean Chew
Denise Dalton	Cheryl Floyd
Gloria Harris	Daryl Lance, Pharma.D.
Alan Lim, M.D.	Therese Nakata
Muriel Oles	Gina Petrak
Linda Reib	Becky Richards, R.N.
Jami Turner	Helene Wolf

Preface

Healing Takes Time

It all began with a concern: a lump was discovered, or your mammogram showed something suspicious. That's the first time the word "cancer" entered your mind. Sure, it happens to everyone. But me?

You start getting anxious; you want answers immediately. But answers often take time. So does a follow-up test, or the results of a biopsy. Initially you weren't concerned, but you are beginning to wonder if everything will be all right.

Then you find out you have breast cancer! What was originally nothing more than a routine annual mammogram has turned into a long and scary journey. Things on your "To Do" list that seemed immensely important only a few days ago have suddenly become irrelevant. New tests are ordered; you now have to wait for *these* results.

At the same time, you have to gather up all of your courage to tell your loved ones—not only that you have breast cancer, but that everything will be okay. (But deep inside you may wonder, will it?) Everyone will want to know what is happening to you, but you don't even know yourself!

STOP!

Take a deep breath. You have time to gather your thoughts, to make informed decisions.

You don't have to become an immediate expert on everything

remotely related to breast cancer. However, it is important to have a general understanding of the disease that is now confronting you, and to fully comprehend the treatment options that are available. This book will help, as will innumerable discussions with your healthcare team in the coming months.

There will be lots of "waiting" throughout your treatment regimen: waiting for the next doctor's appointment; waiting for a return phone call; waiting for lab results. Radiation will start—you can't wait till it ends. Chemotherapy commences. You can't wait to feel better!

With each wait, your anxiety and stress levels increase. You sense a "loss of control," that the treatment is taking over your life.

But it doesn't have to. In fact, *you* are in control—every step of the way. Yes, you have to confront this disease, but you can do so on your own terms.

First, accept the fact that the treatment and recovery process takes time. Answers will come, treatments will succeed. Never as quickly as you would like, but they will.

Second, establish good relationships with your healthcare team—your surgeon, oncologist, radiologist, nurses, social workers and others. Always communicate *any* concerns that you have. Remember that all treatment decisions are *your* decisions.

Finally, establish a support system. This could involve other women who have been through a similar experience, family members, close friends, clergy or social workers. You will soon find that others want to help, *need* to help. Allow them to. You do not have to go through this alone.

It is easy to say, "Just relax and don't worry." But you won't relax—and of course you will worry. Nonetheless, you *will* get through this. It won't be easy at times. But you will. And in some very important ways, you will come out the better for it. You will forever appreciate the simple joys that life affords, and the special people that have always been there for you.

Most importantly, you may discover an extraordinary inner strength that you did not realize you had. As the poet E.E. Cummings once wrote:

"In the midst of winter I suddenly learned
that there was within me an invincible summer!"

Heal well. Stay well!

Ernie Bodai and Richard Zmuda

"I Flunked My Mammogram!"
What you need to know about breast cancer
NOW!

INTRODUCTION

PART I: SCREENING FOR BREAST CANCER

PART III: RECOVERY

APPENDICES

INDEX

Introduction

You've heard the number often enough – "One out of eight women will get breast cancer in their lifetime." Unfortunately, *you* are now that one out of eight. You certainly didn't choose to be, but you are.

As such, here is the statistic that you should *now* focus on: **More than 95 percent of women whose breast cancer is caught in its earliest stages will be healthy and disease-free five years after their diagnosis and treatment**. Even if your breast cancer was not caught early, the outlook is extremely promising. In fact, **the five-year survival rate for ALL women with breast cancer still exceeds 85 percent!**

Major advances in screening mammography, which are just around the corner, will enable us to detect breast tumors at much smaller sizes. New anti-cancer drugs are emerging from clinical trials, and the revolutionary decoding of the human DNA sequence will eventually lead to the elimination of cancer as a life-threatening illness. Cancer may still occur, but it will no longer be the medical challenge that it is today.

You already have at your disposal an extraordinary array of treatments, many of which did not exist a decade ago. Your cancer *can* be beaten. It's not just hype. It's hope, and it's here.

A Breast Cancer Primer

The female breast is primarily made up of skin, fat and connective tissues, with arteries, veins and nerves interspersed throughout. (See Figure I.) Each breast has 15 to 20 sections called *lobes;*

5

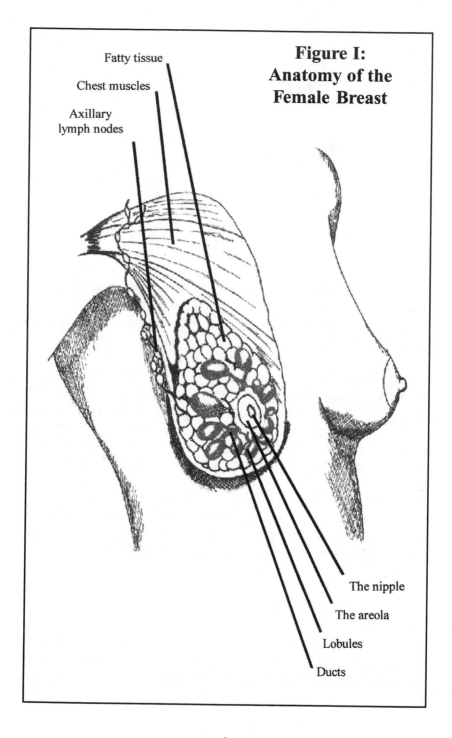

Fatty tissue

Chest muscles

Axillary
lymph nodes

**Figure I:
Anatomy of the
Female Breast**

The nipple

The areola

Lobules

Ducts

each lobe has many smaller sections called *lobules*. The lobules make the breast milk, which is then carried to the nipple through a system of thin tubes called *ducts*. A layer of muscle lies underneath the breast but is not considered part of the breast itself.

The most common type of breast cancer forms in the cells of the ducts and is called *ductal carcinoma*. Cancer that begins in the lobes or lobules is called *lobular carcinoma*. Less commonly, breast cancer can affect the nipple, a condition called *Paget's disease*. Rarely, it can be found primarily in the lymphatic vessels and skin, a condition called *inflammatory breast cancer*.

What exactly is cancer?

The actual word "cancer" is confusing. It is a catch-all term for diseases that are characterized by the uncontrolled growth of cells. The exact type of cancer that you have is categorized by its origin; in your case it is called *breast* cancer because it originated somewhere in the breast (ducts, lobules, etc.) Even if the cancer spreads (*metastasizes*) from the breast to another part of the body, it is still referred to as "breast cancer."

In its simplest terms, a cancer cell is a cell that just doesn't know when or how to stop dividing. All cells have a natural lifespan, but sometimes a cell just won't die when its time is up. The cell may have been altered by some outside factor, or in the case of inherited cancers, a mutation in its genetic code may have been passed down from earlier generations, causing it to keep dividing and growing.

The cancer cell divides into two cancer cells, then four, then eight, and so on. Eventually, there are hundreds and then thousands of them clustering together to form a lump, mass or tumor. It is at this point that it may become detectable with the screening tools we have available today. (See Figure II.)

Cancer doesn't just appear overnight; it takes years to develop to a detectable stage. Once it grows to a certain level, it expands exponentially. If left unchecked, these out-of-control cells eventually spread

Figure II:

Clinical Growth Rate of Breast Cancer

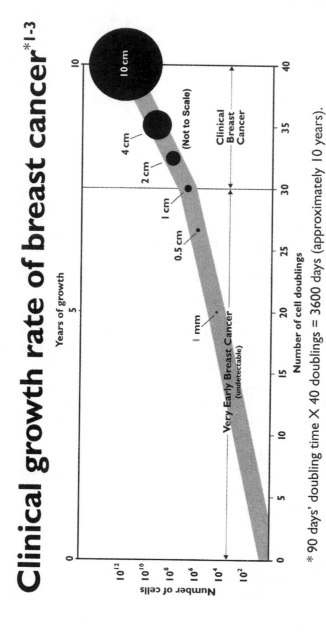

* 90 days' doubling time X 40 doublings = 3600 days (approximately 10 years).

References: 1. Harris JR, Hellman S. Natural history of breast cancer. In: Harris JR, Hellman S, Henderson IC, et al, eds. *Breast Diseases.* 2nd ed. Philadelphia, Pa: JB Lippincott Company; 1991:165-189. **2.** Collins VP, Loeffler RK, Tivey H. Observations on growth rates of human tumors. *Am J Roentgenol.* 1956;76:988-1000. **3.** Fisher B. The evolution of paradigms for the management of breast cancer: a personal perspective. *Cancer Res.* 1992;52:2371-2383.

ZENECA Pharmaceuticals
A Business Unit of Zeneca Inc. Wilmington, Delaware 19850-5437

Roche **Pharmaceuticals**

to nearby tissues, and then to other tissues and organs farther away. While this process usually takes a long time, we are nonetheless in a hurry to treat the disease.

Cancerous cells can spread to other parts of the body in two ways: they can grow into a mass (tumor) and invade nearby tissues or organs; or they can break away and spread through the bloodstream or the *lymphatic* system to other parts of the body. The lymphatic system is composed of many organs dispersed throughout the body; it is responsible for cleansing the blood. Lymph nodes are tiny "filters" that remove toxins and other foreign bodies from surrounding tissues.

Breast lumps or tumors can be *benign* (non-cancerous) or *malignant* (cancerous). A benign tumor can be removed and in most cases will not come back. A malignant tumor, on the other hand, is a collection of cells which grow and can affect nearby tissues or can break away and travel to distant parts of the body. It is important to note that most breast lumps or tumors are not cancerous.

No Single Cause

Only five to ten percent of breast cancers are hereditary; that is, they are caused by a faulty gene that has been passed down from generation to generation. The vast majority of breast cancers are caused by something else—we still don't have a specific clue as to a definitive cause for the disease. Many theories have been proposed, all of which have their supporters.

Take diet, for example. Breast cancer is rare in some populations of women, and their cultural diets may play a role. Japanese women have extremely low rates of breast cancer compared with American women. But when Japanese women emigrate to the United States, their rates of breast cancer soon escalate to the American level. Many researchers theorize that diet may be the culprit; in Japan the typical diet is high in soy and low in fat. Unfortunately, the reverse is true for many American diets, which rarely include soy but have plenty of fat.

Beyond diet, a number of studies have focused on environmental factors, early onset of menstruation, nulliparity (never had a pregnancy), hormone replacement therapy, stress, radiation exposure—the list goes on and on. In fact, breast cancer is likely the result of a combination of factors.

* * * * *

Having said all of this, here you are—either facing a significant risk of breast cancer, or possibly having just been diagnosed. You may even be on the welcome road to recovery.

Whatever the reason, you now have this book in your hands and have therefore taken an important first step. We are going to help you take many more.

My Notes

"Initial Questions That I Have"
(Things I just don't understand yet!)

_____

_____

_____

_____

_____

_____

_____

_____

_____

_____

_____

_____

_____

PART I:

Screening for Breast Cancer

Risk Factors

"I already HAVE breast cancer," you might say. "So why should I worry about risk factors NOW?"

On the surface, it does seem rather silly. However, unless you have a strong family history of breast cancer, you may never know exactly what caused your cancer. Therefore, as you move beyond treatment and recovery toward a long and healthy life, you will clearly want to do everything you can to minimize the risk of the cancer coming back (*recurring*) or developing in the other breast.

A recent survey of European women with breast cancer found that only nine percent of them believed that an unhealthy diet contributed to their disease. Yet nearly a third of the women significantly changed their dietary habits after their diagnosis. Why? The better question is, why not?

Many of the women reduced their consumption of fat, sugar and red meat; they began eating more fruits and vegetables and started taking vitamin supplements. This was especially true for younger women. The researchers suggested that these dietary changes represented a way for women to exert some form of influence over their own well-being.

They were right! Keep in mind that you *always* have some influence over factors affecting not only your cancer risk, but also your overall health. As these women would tell you, it simply can't hurt to improve your diet, exercise more, and generally take better care of yourself.

Such changes will have benefits far beyond reducing your risk factors for cancer. You'll feel stronger, healthier, have a more positive outlook on life, and possibly avoid dozens of *other* ailments that directly result from an unhealthy lifestyle.

What about a family history of breast cancer, something that is totally out of your control? Does that put you at greater risk? Yes, it definitely does. But what if you have *no* history of breast cancer in your family. Does that mean that you are off the hook? Unfortunately, no.

About three-quarters of newly diagnosed breast cancer patients have no known history of the disease in their family. Keep in mind that the last generation often did not discuss sensitive issues such as breast cancer, and important diagnostic tests were not available 20 or 30 years ago. Many of us, therefore, may have had a close relative with breast cancer, but simply have no knowledge of it.

Diet

There are Asian diets rich in soy; olive oil-laden Mediterranean diets; low-fat diets; vegetarian diets. Wow! The headlines are full of stories touting the newest cancer-fighting cuisines.

In all likelihood, diet may play a role in the onset of some cancers, including breast cancer. Results from several major studies have shown that the rates of breast cancer in certain countries are far lower than those in the United States. Is a healthier diet the reason? Or is it the consumption of certain culture-specific foods? Studies to date have not been conclusive, yet the data appear to be far too convincing to ignore.

For example, take Asian/Pacific Islander women. Large-scale studies have noted the sharply lower rates of breast cancer for these women in their native countries, as compared with much higher rates for Asian/Pacific Islander immigrants—and their descendants—in the United States.

Studies have shown that breast cancer rates for these women increase significantly once they begin living in the United States. The risk increases even further for second and third generations residing in the U.S.

(Interestingly, back in Japan, traditionally low breast cancer rates are now increasing at a significant pace. Is this the result of the gradual "Westernization" of Japanese society? Nobody knows for sure.)

The reasons for the increased risk of breast cancer among immigrant women who come to the United States remain elusive. Western diets, high in polyunsaturated fat, could be a factor. Fat intake may lead to higher levels of the hormone estradiol, an estrogen that has been linked to an increased breast cancer risk.

Unfortunately, obesity is at an all-time high in the United States. This unhealthy situation may be responsible for *many* health-related problems, including a higher rate of breast cancer. According to the American Obesity Association, 22 percent of the total adult U.S. population—39 million people—meet the criteria for obesity.

Whether you have cancer or not, a healthier diet that is low in fat and high in fruits and vegetables is a great first step toward minimizing the risk of breast cancer or its recurrence. And why not throw in a little soy or olive oil in the process? It certainly can't hurt, and it may taste good too!

Genetic Risk

Genes are the basic units of heredity—affecting traits or characteristics that are passed down from generation to generation. They determine obvious traits, such as facial features, eye and hair color, as well as more subtle ones, such as the oxygen-carrying ability of blood. It is estimated that humans have approximately 100,000 genes, but a flaw in *any one* of them could result in some specific disease.

In 1994, researchers from the National Institutes of Health were studying three families of Ashkenazi Jews that had an extremely strong history of breast cancer. The families were not known to be related, but they each carried an identical defect (*mutation*) on a specific gene that the researchers called BRCA1 (BReast CAncer 1). Every person carries this gene, but most do not have the mutated version.

In recent years, scientists have identified an additional gene—BRCA2—which, along with BRCA1, seems to account for the majority of *inherited* cases of breast cancer. **However, only five to ten percent of breast cancer cases are caused by this type of inherited, genetic defect.** If you test positive for the 'gene,' it means that there is an 80 percent chance that you will get breast cancer by the time you reach the age of 80. It does not mean that you will get breast cancer right away, but your *lifetime* risk is definitely increased.

A blood test is now available to determine whether a woman carries a mutated BRCA1 or BRCA2 gene. However, even if a woman has a family history of breast cancer, or is associated with a higher-risk ethnic population, the value of genetic testing remains controversial.

If a woman tests positive for the breast cancer gene, she will undoubtedly have many emotional issues to cope with. Not only would a positive genetic test be of concern to her, but it would also have implications for her family members as well. Should sisters be tested? How will *they* cope? Should daughters be tested? At what age?

In addition, would information from genetic testing remain confidential? Because current laws protecting a patient's medical privacy are not foolproof, the potential for employment and insurance discrimination exists.

What should you do with this information? Should you have a bilateral prophylactic mastectomy to remove both breasts before cancer occurs? Should you take tamoxifen, a drug with potentially significant side effects, to try to prevent the development of breast cancer? We are not sure.

However, if you have already had genetic testing and a BRCA marker has been identified, it is important that you speak with a professional genetic counselor. Such knowledgeable support may be invaluable in helping you—and your family members—make informed decisions.

Hormones

Estrogen is the major female hormone, produced primarily by the ovaries. It aids in developing female sex organs and in regulating monthly menstrual cycles. *Progesterone* is a hormone that is released by the ovaries during every menstrual cycle. It helps to prepare a woman's body for pregnancy.

After a woman goes through menopause, her production of these hormones falls drastically. In the short term, hot flashes, bone loss, vaginal dryness and mood swings can occur. In the long term, a woman faces a greater risk of osteoporosis (weakening of the bones), heart disease, stroke and Alzheimer's disease.

Hormone replacement therapy—often referred to as HRT—is used to replace the hormones no longer being produced after menopause. HRT can significantly reduce a woman's risk of osteoporosis and heart disease. While developing breast cancer is a major concern, up to 10 times as many women die from vascular disease each year than from breast cancer. The use of HRT, therefore, is a very important consideration for all postmenopausal women.

Yet exposure to hormones is believed to increase a woman's risk of developing breast cancer. Since HRT adds estrogen (and often progesterone) back to the body, many studies have looked for a possible link between the use of HRT and breast cancer.

Although it has yet to be proven that estrogen *causes* breast cancer, estrogen may help some breast cancer cells grow when the tumor is *already present* in your body. (This is a good example of why risk factors are important, even after the diagnosis of cancer.)

Therefore, once a diagnosis of breast cancer is made, tests

will be done to see if the cancer is "positive" for estrogen and progesterone receptors. These receptors are the parts of the cell that attract these hormones. They may help the cancerous cells to grow—something we don't want.

If the cancer is found to have these receptors, estrogen and progesterone can attach themselves to breast cancer cells and stimulate their growth. In such cases, anti-hormone therapies, such as tamoxifen, can be used to prevent damaging hormones from further stimulating the cancer cells to grow.

Recent studies indicate that using only estrogen for HRT is acceptable, but adding progesterone to the mix is not. In other words, there seems to be a significantly increased risk if hormone replacement therapy includes a combination of *both* estrogen and progesterone, as opposed to using estrogen by itself.

Estrogen given alone, by contrast, is known to increase the incidence of uterine cancer. Is all this confusing? That's certainly understandable, especially since there is no consensus among medical professionals themselves.

In considering hormone replacement therapy, you need to evaluate your own individual risk for osteoporosis and heart disease, and weigh it against your risk for developing breast cancer. Also, menopausal symptoms affect different people in different ways. If the symptoms are significantly affecting your quality of life, HRT may be the right choice. If you are sailing through menopause with only minor or fleeting symptoms, HRT may not be necessary. Talk to your doctor to find out whether hormone replacement therapy is appropriate for you.

Race

We have mentioned that Asians have a lower risk of breast cancer and Ashkenazi Jews have a higher risk. What of African Americans and Hispanics? African Americans have a lower incidence of breast cancer than Caucasians, but a higher mortality. Why? We don't know, but it has been shown that breast cancer appears to be more aggressive and is often diagnosed at a more advanced stage in African-American women.

Hispanics, similarly, have a lower incidence of breast cancer, but have mortality rates approaching those in the African-American community. Screening rates are lower for Hispanic women, particularly in terms of breast self-exams. It may be that religious beliefs, particularly in Hispanic and Hindu women, among others, discourage breast self-examination. These women often do not feel comfortable with "touching" themselves. Because of the importance of breast self-exam, such feelings of guilt need to be dispelled.

Additional Factors

The headlines are constantly touting the cancer-fighting properties of this fruit or that vegetable, or telling us of a new "breast cancer risk factor" that has just been identified.

Hundreds of ongoing studies are focusing on an extraordinary number of potential risk factors: an early first menstrual period; late menopause; exposure to pesticides and electromagnetic fields; lack of physical activity; anxiety and depression; alcohol consumption; even eating flame-broiled foods!

But the fact remains that the majority of breast cancers have no single, identifiable risk factor that can be pinpointed as a definitive cause. What's a woman to do? You can't change your family history or heritage. But you can change to a low-fat diet; watch your weight; get plenty of exercise; and stop stressing about the little things in life.

Be wary of claims that super-high doses of certain vitamins or herbs will stave off breast cancer or prevent its return. In fact, excessive amounts of many of these supplements can be dangerous, especially if taken over a prolonged period. Common sense—rather than uncommon measures–should be the yardstick used for minimizing your breast cancer risk.

The Gail Model

In 1990, Dr. Mitchell Gail, a researcher from the National Cancer Institute, developed a mathematical model to help predict breast cancer risk. The Gail Model incorporates seven key factors: age, race, number of first degree relatives with a history of breast cancer, age at first live birth, age at menarche (first period), number of breast biopsies, and a history of atypical hyperplasia.

Although it has been modified somewhat over the past decade, the Gail Model is still the predominant tool used to determine breast cancer risk for women in the general population. Importantly, it is also a major guideline used for enrolling patients in the Study of Tamoxifen and Raloxifene (STAR) clinical trial. (See page 26.)

My Notes

"My Personal Risk Factors"
(Which ones can I minimize?)

_____

_____

_____

_____

_____

_____

_____

_____

_____

_____

_____

_____

_____

_____

Prevention?

Can breast cancer be prevented? Not yet, and maybe never. But we can certainly minimize a number of risk factors for the disease, especially with a low-fat, high fruit and vegetable diet, and getting plenty of exercise.

Beyond these important self-help measures, there are also some promising research initiatives that may bring us closer to this elusive goal. An extremely important clinical trial is taking place (the STAR trial, discussed shortly), which is testing two drugs that have been shown to dramatically lower the risk of breast cancer in women believed to be at high risk of developing the disease.

Some women with a strong family history of breast cancer may also consider the option of prophylactic mastectomy—removing their healthy breasts when there is no sign of cancer—in an effort to reduce the risk of the disease. The physical, emotional and psychological impacts of such a decision are significant.

A number of researchers are also focusing on specific vitamins and minerals that—when consumed in high doses—appear to have a cancer-preventive effect. Other researchers are developing "cancer vaccines" that may have the same revolutionary success as the polio vaccines of yesteryear and the measles vaccines of today.

For now, though, there is no sure-fire way to actually *prevent* breast cancer. Someday, maybe. But not yet.

Exercise

Studies have shown that regular exercise—even 30 minutes, 2 to 3 times a week—can lower estrogen levels. (Estrogen has been linked to breast cancer risk.) In addition, fat cells store estrogen, so the less fat you carry, the less estrogen you store—and the less potential stimulation of breast cancer cells.

Additional benefits of exercise include increased lung capacity, muscle strength and overall energy levels. You'll feel more in control, have higher self-esteem, and experience less anxiety and depression. While there will be times during your treatment and recovery when it may be difficult for you to exercise, even a minimal exercise schedule can be tailored to your individual needs.

Some researchers believe that as many as one-third of all breast cancer cases could be related to lack of exercise and a poor diet—highly preventable risk factors! And yet almost two-thirds of American adults remain inactive, despite the long list of well-known health benefits.

Exercise is a healthy choice to pursue for many reasons, not the least of which is the possibility of reducing breast cancer risk.

The STAR Trial

A large clinical trial was launched by the National Cancer Institute in 1999 to see which of two major breast cancer drugs—tamoxifen or raloxifene—might work better to reduce the incidence of breast cancer, or possibly *prevent* the disease. The Study of Tamoxifen and Raloxifene (STAR) will eventually enroll 22,000 postmenopausal women (women who have gone through menopause) who are at high risk for the disease.

Increased risk of breast cancer is determined in one of two ways. The risk for most women is determined by a computer calculation based on age, number of first-degree relatives with breast cancer, number of suspicious breast biopsies, and other factors per the Gail Model. (See page 22.)

Also, women diagnosed as having lobular carcinoma in situ

(LCIS), a condition that is not cancer but indicates an increased chance of developing invasive breast cancer, are eligible based on that diagnosis alone.

Tamoxifen is a drug taken in pill form that interferes with the activity of estrogen, effectively countering that hormone's cancer-promoting effects. Tamoxifen has been used to treat both early- and advanced-stage breast cancers for more than 20 years. But recent studies have shown that it also dramatically lowers the *incidence* of breast cancer.

Raloxifene is a drug similar to tamoxifen; it is also in pill form. It is being included in the STAR trial based on a surprise finding in a separate study on osteoporosis. Researchers noticed that raloxifene not only reduced the risk of bone fractures in postmenopausal women, but the drug also had a dramatic reduction in the incidence of breast cancer.

While both of these drugs show exceptional promise as breast cancer "preventives," they do have side effects. Those experienced most often by women include hot flashes and other menopausal symptoms such as vaginal discharge, dryness or itching, and painful intercourse.

Women taking tamoxifen were found to have an increased chance of developing three relatively rare conditions: endometrial cancer (cancer of the lining of the uterus), pulmonary embolism (blood clots in the lung), and deep vein thrombosis (blood clots in a major leg vein).

Although women taking raloxifene in clinical trials also demonstrated an increased chance of developing a pulmonary embolism or deep vein thrombosis, the drug did not increase the risk of endometrial cancer.

Importantly, a number of recent studies have found that tamoxifen may have a limited time period for its positive benefits. Researchers have found that taking tamoxifen for ten years was no better than taking it for five years. In fact, some studies have suggested that after five years, tamoxifen can actually begin acting *like* estrogen rather than blocking its effects. Too much of a good thing? Apparently so.

Will tamoxifen and raloxifene be the "magic pills" for preventing breast cancer? No. But hopefully they will be found to have a dramatic impact on *reducing the risk* for many women. In a few years, the STAR trial may let us know for sure.

The National Cancer Institute will be enrolling participants in the STAR trial for a number of years. It is especially intent on reaching out to minority women who traditionally have been underrepresented in major clinical trials. If you are interested in getting more information about the STAR trial, you can call the NCI's Cancer Information Service at 1-800-4CANCER (1-800-422-6237).

Prophylactic Mastectomy

Prophylactic ("preventive") mastectomy involves the removal of one or both healthy breasts when there is no sign of cancer. The procedure is a major operation that is usually followed by immediate (simultaneous) breast reconstruction. It is a drastic alternative undertaken by women who consider themselves to be at very high risk for the disease.

While prophylactic *bilateral* mastectomy (removing *both* breasts) appears to be effective, it remains extremely controversial. Women who are high risk and are considering the procedure are usually given at least two other options: very careful monitoring (which most women choose), and "chemoprevention" with tamoxifen.

(Keep in mind that if breast cancer is caught early, it is highly curable. Careful monitoring, therefore, is an acceptable alternative.)

Prophylactic mastectomy is clearly both a major medical decision and a highly emotional one. Yet among those women who decide to undergo the procedure, most do not appear to have subsequent regrets. They viewed their risk for breast cancer as extremely life-threatening and made their decision accordingly, and comfortably.

A study by researchers at the Mayo Clinic in Rochester, Minnesota found that 70 percent of women who had a bilateral (both breasts) prophylactic mastectomy were satisfied with their decision. Two-thirds of them would likely choose to have the procedure again. Three-quarters of the women said that they are now less concerned about developing breast cancer.

But does it work? Does prophylactic mastectomy actually prevent breast cancer? It probably does. Bilateral prophylactic mastectomy can reduce the risk of breast cancer by up to 90 percent in women at high risk. But it is still not foolproof, and the personal, physical and emotional tradeoffs are significant. It is a decision that requires careful consideration.

Preventing Cancer with Vitamins and Minerals

Studies have shown that more than half of U.S. adults over the age of 65 are taking vitamins with the specific aim of *preventing cancer,* (as are a quarter of those aged 55 to 64). However, while eating plenty of fresh fruits and vegetables has been shown in several studies to possibly lower the risk of developing cancer, there is no convincing evidence that taking just vitamin and mineral supplements provides the same benefits. Neither approach is definitive.

There is little doubt that many dietary supplements, when taken in appropriate doses, can provide healthy benefits. The role they might play in preventing cancer, however, has not been sufficiently researched.

Garlic is a great example. Substances found in garlic have been shown to fight cancer in a test tube but, so far, there is no significant evidence that they can do the same in humans. Yet, how many ads for garlic have you seen on TV, in newspapers, magazines, and so on. Are these claims substantiated? We wish they were, but as of to-day, they are not.

Most vitamin and mineral supplements are not harmful if taken in appropriate doses—and many may certainly have some benefit. But broad claims that a specific vitamin or mineral supplement can single-handedly prevent cancer from occurring are clearly unsubstantiated.

There is real concern that excessive doses of many of these supplements could, in fact, be harmful. For example, vitamin A has been linked to an increased risk of stomach cancer, and concerns have been raised about the interaction of St. John's Wort with certain medi-cines.

Some supplements may skew the results of laboratory tests. Others may alter bleeding times—an important consideration if you are about to undergo surgery. Be sure to disclose to your physician any supplements that you are taking on a regular basis.

Cancer Vaccines

Some pioneering cancer researchers are currently working to develop vaccines that will encourage the body's immune system to recognize cancer cells, just as traditional vaccines for mumps and measles target those infectious diseases.

Vaccines work by exposing your body's immune system to a weakened version of the specific disease. This then stimulates your immune system to produce cells called *antibodies* to fight the unwel-come invaders. Once your body has produced antibodies for a spe-cific disease, it can remember how to recognize them in the future. In terms of cancer, these antibodies may destroy any cancer cells that develop, or at least slow their growth.

The manufacture of vaccines against specific cancers is a very promising avenue of cancer research. Such vaccines could be used either as preventive treatments to stop people from actually getting cancer, or could be used together with traditional cancer-fighting treatments (surgery, radiation, chemotherapy) to target existing or recurrent tumors.

While the practical use of vaccines to prevent and treat cancer may still be years away, dramatic advances in our understanding of the human genetic code could move that timetable up significantly.

Risk Reduction

While cancer cannot be "prevented," your risk for the disease or its recurrence may well be minimized. Significant risk *reduction*, rather than prevention, is an achievable goal. And *major* risk reduction is certainly within your personal capability. Researchers are doing their part and making remarkable strides. So can you!

Screening Techniques

Without a doubt, early detection is the key to having many more treatment options at your disposal—and it gives you a better chance for an excellent outcome. The best way to do this is through regular breast cancer screening.

Most women who think of screening for breast cancer think of mammograms. But there are actually *three* ways to screen for breast cancer that, when combined, offer the best opportunity to detect the disease at its earliest, most treatable stage. These are:

- Breast self-exam (BSE);
- Clinical breast exam (CBE) by a healthcare professional;
- Mammography.

Most healthcare organizations recommend the following minimum screening guidelines:

- Perform a monthly breast self-exam beginning at age 20.
- Have a clinical breast exam by a healthcare professional at least every 3 years beginning at age 20, and yearly after age 35.
- Have a baseline mammogram at age 35, and yearly after age 40.

These recommendations apply to those women who are at "normal risk" and do not develop intervening symptoms, such as the finding of a new lump, which calls for immediate attention.

Breast Self-Exam

You know *your* breasts. For that reason alone, breast self-exam (see Figure III) is the most important long-term screening strategy for

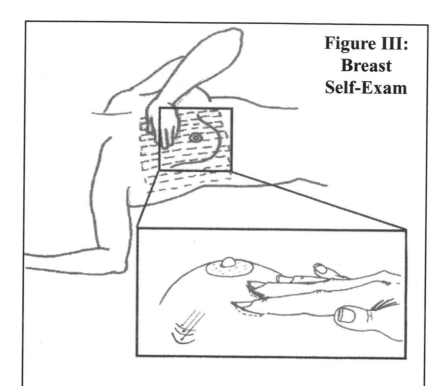

**Figure III:
Breast
Self-Exam**

Three Steps to a Complete Breast Self-Exam

1. Lie down and place a pillow under your right shoulder. Put your right hand above your head. With the fingertips of your left hand use small circles and up-and-down motions to check your entire right breast. Use three different levels of pressure: soft, medium and hard. Repeat this for the left side.

2. Look in a mirror for any changes in the shape of your breasts and check for dimpling. Note any nipple discharge, but do not squeeze your nipples.

3. In the shower, raise your right arm. Then with the soapy fingertips of your left hand use small circles and up-and-down motions to check your entire right breast. Repeat this for your left breast.

breast cancer. Check your breasts regularly—at the same time each month—in a careful, consistent way. *Unfortunately, the vast majority of women simply don't bother. Or, if they do, they do it incorrectly.*

While it may sound strange, take the time to become "familiar with your breasts." You may be surprised to find out how naturally lumpy they are! Over the course of the first few months of breast self-exams, you will get to know the normal feel of your breasts. Then you will be ready to watch for any unusual changes that might take place. Any change should be reported to your physician.

It is important to perform breast self-exams at the same time each month, preferably at the end of each menstrual cycle. This is when your hormonal levels will be at their lowest, thus exerting a minimal influence on your breast tissue. Menstruation can also affect the tenderness, fullness and lumpiness of your breasts.

Always perform your breast self-exam in the same, consistent way so you will notice any changes or "differences" in the tissues. Your doctor will not expect you to say that you have a suspicious finding. He or she will only expect you to report that something is new or different.

Clinical Breast Exam

A clinical breast exam is a thorough physical examination of your breasts by a medical professional. It involves a doctor or nurse looking at and feeling the entire breast and chest area, including the lymph nodes above and below the collarbone and under each arm.

It is important that you have both your mammogram and clinical breast exam done closely together. Don't put these appointments off! Fifteen to 20 percent of all breast cancers may go undetected by relying on a mammogram alone. Make it an annual event, perhaps tied to your birthday. It could be your present to yourself. *It could save your life!*

A Primer on Mammograms

A mammogram is simply an x-ray taken of the breast. The purpose of a *screening* mammogram is to look for anything unusual when you do not have any specific problems or concerns. (A *diagnostic* mammogram is a more detailed, follow-up look at something that seemed suspicious on the screening mammogram.)

Mammography is not perfect, but it is still the best screening tool available today. A mammogram is able to detect breast cancer *years* before it becomes large enough to be felt.

A mammogram can be done in a doctor's office, a hospital clinic or even a mobile van. It involves an x-ray picture taken by a technologist, which is then carefully reviewed by a radiologist to check for cancer or other breast changes.

To get a good picture, the technologist will need to compress your breasts, sometimes to a point of discomfort. It only lasts a few seconds, and the discomfort is well worth the increased accuracy obtained by getting a good mammographic examination. (New products, such as Biolucent's foam cushion MammoPad®, can significantly reduce this discomfort.)

Ensuring a Quality Mammogram

In 1992, Congress enacted the Mammography Quality Standards Act (MQSA) which requires the Food and Drug Administration to certify that mammography facilities are safe and reliable. To find an FDA-approved mammography facility near you, or to check the certification status of the facility you currently use, call 1-800-4-CAN-CER. The FDA has also established a website at www.fda.gov/cdrh/mammography/consumers.

Once you find a facility, don't hesitate to ask what percentage of their time is spent on mammograms, and if they have a radiologist who specializes in mammography. Far from being offended, a quality clinic will welcome such inquiries—and be proud of their level of expertise.

False-Positive Mammograms

You may have heard about so-called "false-positive" mammograms. A false-positive result from a mammogram means that something looked suspicious and you were called back for additional testing, but in the end nothing abnormal was found.

Needless to say, a false-positive result—a false alarm, if you will—can be a very scary experience.

If you have regular screening mammograms throughout your life, there is a chance that at some point you will have an incorrect, false-positive result. Why do false-positives occur? Basically, because mammograms—and the radiologists who read them—are not perfect.

You are more likely to get a misinterpreted (false-positive) mammogram if you are younger; have denser breast tissue; have a family history of breast cancer; have used estrogen; or if there has been a long interval between mammograms.

Try to have your mammogram performed at a clinic that specializes in mammography, rather than at an x-ray facility where the technicians are more attuned to broken bones than breast abnormalities. As with any skill, the more frequently a person performs a particular task, the more expert they become.

Breast cancer experts agree that the number of false positives—and thus unnecessary follow-up procedures such as additional mammograms and biopsies—must be reduced. However, **don't let that deter you from getting an annual mammogram!** The risk of cancer going undetected far outweighs the short-term anxiety of receiving a false-positive test result.

The technology of mammography is changing rapidly—and

for the better. The new techniques becoming available can locate much smaller tumors, especially in dense breast tissue. They can also more accurately determine whether the tumors are cancerous or not, thus avoiding the need for additional diagnostic tests or biopsies.

Furthermore, many of these new technologies are taking much of the human guesswork out of the process. The possibility of diagnostic error by a radiologist is being minimized by increasingly detailed images from computers and mammogram machines.

Calcifications or Calcium Deposits

Small white specks called *calcifications* often appear on a mammogram. Calcifications are tiny mineral deposits within the breast tissue or arteries. They are divided into two categories: *macro*calcifications and *micro*calcifications (*macro* meaning large, *micro* meaning small).

*Macro*calcifications are larger, coarse calcium deposits that likely represent benign (non-cancerous) changes in the breast due to aging of the breast arteries, old injuries, or inflammation. Macrocalcifications are found in about 50 percent of women over the age of 50, and in about 10 percent of women under age 50.

*Micro*calcifications are much smaller calcium deposits in the breast; they can indicate the presence of early cancer. The shape and arrangement of these microcalcifications are very important in helping the radiologist judge the likelihood of disease.

Recent studies have shown that calcium deposits in *arteries* in the breast—called breast arterial calcifications or BACs—might also indicate that there are additional calcium deposits within the coronary (heart) arteries. This could serve as an important early warning sign for heart disease—another bonus from getting an annual mammogram! (Remember, more women die from coronary heart disease than from breast cancer.)

Ductal Lavage

A relatively new technique, *ductal lavage*, is being studied as a potential additional measure for breast cancer screening. With ductal lavage, a physician places a catheter into a duct, injects a small amount of saline, and then removes the fluid to examine cells that line the milk ducts inside the breast. Since breast cancer often starts in these cells, it is a logical first place to look for suspicious, atypical cells that might eventually become cancerous.

There exist many problems with the technique. It can be uncomfortable for the patient, examination of the cells can be complicated, and while it has been touted as a "screening technique," its results for early detection of breast cancer are dismal, at best.

Even if an analysis of the fluid shows the presence of abnormal cells, it may be difficult to actually locate the cancer. Ductal lavage has shown some promise in clinical trials, especially for women considered at high risk for breast cancer, but it is not currently considered accurate enough to be used as a standard screening technique.

Diagnostic Procedures

What if something suspicious or abnormal appears on your screening mammogram? Or a new lump is detected through a breast self-exam or clinical breast exam? There are a number of follow-up diagnostic procedures that may be performed to take a closer look.

A **diagnostic mammogram** is a more detailed mammogram than the one used for screening purposes. It involves a number of different images of the breast, focusing in greater detail on the area that appeared suspicious on the screening mammogram.

Ultrasound uses high-frequency sound waves to evaluate a suspicious breast lump. It can be ordered as an additional study and can be particularly helpful if a woman has dense breast tissue, which is much more common in younger women.

Scintimammography is an imaging technique that uses radioactive tracers given as an injection. These tracers travel through the bloodstream and eventually settle in the breast, where they concentrate in cancer cells. The tracers are then picked up on a computer image. Scintimammography is particularly effective with dense breast tissue, implants, previous surgeries (biopsies), and after radiation therapy.

Digital mammography takes a digital image of the breast instead of using film as in traditional mammography. (This is similar to the distinction between film and digital photography.) Digital images have several distinct advantages: they are available in seconds, provide better resolution than mammograms, and they can be stored or sent electronically.

Computer-Aided Detection (CAD) systems such as the ImageChecker® (R2 Technology) scan digital images of a mammogram and mark areas on the image where the computer finds a pattern suggestive of an early cancer. The radiologist can then focus on these suspicious areas for further evaluation.

Magnetic resonance imaging (MRI) is a technique which uses magnetic fields to excite particles in soft tissues, thereby creating an image or picture. It is capable of detecting some changes missed by conventional mammography and may be useful in staging. It is the technique of choice if one is concerned that a breast implant may have ruptured.

Positron emission tomography (PET) scanning looks not at the structures themselves but rather at the activity going on within them. For breast cancer, PET scanning looks at how much glucose (sugar) is being used by breast tissues. A higher level of the sugar molecule uptake indicates that these cells may have higher energy requirements, a characteristic of many cancer cells.

A **biopsy** may also be recommended. A *biopsy* means the removal of tissue for closer inspection under a microscope. There are several different types of biopsies, including fine needle aspiration, core biopsy, needle localization biopsy, stereotactic core biopsy, and an open surgical biopsy.

A **fine needle aspiration** uses a slender needle to remove fluid or suspicious tissue from a breast lump. The sample is then sent to a pathologist to check for cancerous cells.

A **core biopsy** uses a larger needle to remove a piece of suspicious tissue from the breast. Sometimes mammography or ultrasonography is used to help guide the needle. The tissue is then sent to a pathologist to check for cancerous cells.

A **needle localization biopsy** involves inserting a thin needle into the breast to find the exact area of concern. A wire is then passed through the needle to the area that will be biopsied. Sometimes mammography or ultrasonography is used to help guide the needle. In addition, blue dye may be injected into the area to help in localizing the mass. An open surgical biopsy is then performed, and the sample is sent for pathology analysis.

A **stereotactic core biopsy** uses a stereotactic biopsy machine to remove suspicious tissue for examination under a microscope. A mammogram and a computer are used to guide the biopsy needle, which can take multiple samples that are then sent to a pathologist.

Finally, an **open surgical biopsy** involves a surgeon removing part or all of the lump or suspicious area. The sample is then sent to a pathologist to check for cancerous cells.

One minimally-invasive alternative to open surgical biopsy is the **Mammotome®** (Ethicon Endo-Surgery, Johnson & Johnson), which is a hand-held biopsy device that involves no stitches and can be used in a doctor's office. The Mammotome® is used in conjunction with a stereotactic biopsy machine or ultrasound. Through a unique vacuum-assisted technique, it appears to provide accurate samples for a wide variety of breast abnormalities. In fact, it can often completely remove small cancers.

If any biopsy tests come back positive—that is, cancer has been detected—additional tests may be needed to see if the tumor is sensitive to estrogen or progesterone, or to determine the aggressiveness of the tumor. These additional tests will be done on the tissue that was removed, without any further discomfort to you. They are necessary to plan the best type of treatment.

The pathology report may classify the tumor according to the 9-point Bloom Richardson Scale or BR Scale, which evaluates tumors based on three factors: the ability of the cells to form tubular structures; the size and shape of the cancer cells; and the number of dividing cells.

A BR score of 3-5 indicates a Grade I (low grade, less aggressive) tumor; 6-7 represents a Grade II (intermediate) tumor; 8-9 is a Grade III (high grade) tumor. The BR score is an important factor in determing the most appropriate treatment strategy.

Minority Screening

More Caucasian women are having mammograms than ever before—about three-fourths of those over age 50. In 1987, only 27 percent of women in that age group reported having had a mammogram. That overall success rate, however, has not been realized outside of Caucasian, heterosexual women.

For example, American-Asian and Pacific Islander women have one of the lowest breast and cervical cancer screening rates of all ethnic groups in the United States. Nearly one-third of the women in these groups have *never* had a mammogram. The rates are particularly dismal for Asian-Hindu women, more than two-thirds of whom have never had a mammogram.

Similar studies document significantly lower screening rates for African-American and Hispanic women, as compared with Caucasian women. Other studies have shown that lesbians have mammograms at approximately half the rate of heterosexual women.

It also appears that *income level* may play a role in mammography screening rates; fewer than half of women below the federal poverty level have an annual mammogram. Yet there are programs in place to provide free or discounted mammograms, and many insurance programs, including Medicare and Medicaid, may provide coverage for screening mammograms.

For more information, ask your healthcare provider or call the Cancer Information Service at 1-800-4CANCER. Breast cancer is a highly treatable disease, especially if caught early. That makes it even more tragic when important screening opportunities are not provided to those most in need of them.

Benign (Non-Cancerous) Breast Changes

All women experience changes in their breasts from time to time. Most commonly, fluctuating hormone levels during the menstrual cycle can cause changes in the look, feel and tenderness of your breasts. If there are any unusual breast changes that are long-lasting or cause you concern, make an appointment with your physician. Most of these conditions will prove to be normal and not cancerous.

Breast Pain

Breast pain is extremely common—two out of three women suffer from breast pain at some time in their lives. Like any other breast problem, the pain can be worrisome, but breast pain is rarely the only indicator of an underlying breast cancer. If you have persistent breast pain, however, or pain associated with a lump, you should see your doctor.

There are two types of breast pain: pain related to the menstrual cycle (cyclical), and pain unrelated to your cycle (non-cyclical). Most frequently, breast pain is associated with normal changes in hormonal levels during the menstrual cycle, or possibly the presence of a non-cancerous breast cyst (fluid-filled sac). It often disappears as mysteriously as it appears. Medical treatment for breast pain will depend upon the cause.

Fibrocystic Changes

This term applies to the generalized lumpiness of the breast. Women sometimes describe the lumpiness as "ropy" or "granular." Cysts may also be present. Frequently cysts enlarge and become tender or painful just before your period.

Having lumpy breasts is perfectly normal for nearly all women. The most common "lump" is a diffuse nodularity, where the breasts feel generally knobby but without any single outstanding lump. This is part of the normal breast structure and can occur at any time in life, though it tends to happen less after menopause.

Often these changes vary with your menstrual cycle, increasing before a period and decreasing thereafter, and they may be painful. Therefore, make sure to check at the same time each month.

Fibroadenomas

Secondary only to cysts, a fibroadenoma is the most common non-cancerous breast lump. Fibroadenomas can be made of fibrous or glandular tissue. They are somewhat round, soft and moveable.

Fine-needle aspiration or ultrasound may be used to further evaluate these lumps. Many surgeons prefer to surgically remove fibroadenomas, if for no other reason than to simply verify that the lump is benign.

Atypical Hyperplasia

Atypical hyperplasia is a condition in which there are a larger number of breast cells than normal. Also, some of these cells have atypical (unusual) features. This is a non-cancerous (benign) condition, although women with atypical hyperplasia have a higher risk of developing breast cancer in the future.

Nipple Discharge

Nipple discharge is usually not associated with breast cancer. It can be caused by birth control pills or other medications such as sedatives and tranquilizers. Many women who have children continue to have a very slight, milky discharge from both nipples, which may continue for months after breast-feeding stops. Other women with fibrocystic changes may experience a sticky discharge that is brown or green. These are uniformly benign, especially if the discharge occurs from both breasts.

Pre-Cancerous Breast Conditions

Some breast conditions are actually considered *pre-cancerous* or *very early cancers*. These are called "carcinoma in situ." There are two types: lobular carcinoma in situ (LCIS), and ductal carcinoma in situ (DCIS). (See Figure IV.)

Each breast has 15 to 20 overlapping sections called lobes. Within each lobe are many smaller lobules, which end in dozens of tiny bulbs that produce milk. *Lobular* carcinoma in situ (LCIS) arises in these lobules.

The lobes, lobules, and bulbs within the breast are all linked by thin tubes called ducts. These ducts lead to the nipple in the center of a dark area of skin called the areola. *Ductal* carcinoma in situ (DCIS) begins in the lining of these ducts.

LCIS and DCIS have not yet broken through the lobules and ducts to invade the surrounding tissue of the breast to become truly invasive breast cancers. (They are still in place, or *in situ*.)

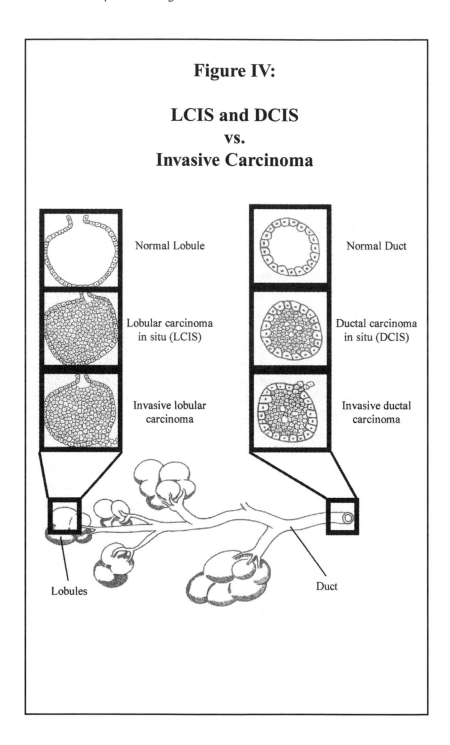

Figure IV:

LCIS and DCIS
vs.
Invasive Carcinoma

Normal Lobule

Normal Duct

Lobular carcinoma
in situ (LCIS)

Ductal carcinoma
in situ (DCIS)

Invasive lobular
carcinoma

Invasive ductal
carcinoma

Lobules

Duct

Lobular Carcinoma In Situ (LCIS)

Lobular carcinoma in situ (LCIS) is rarely seen on a mammogram; it is usually discovered by a breast biopsy done to evaluate another suspicious area. LCIS is not cancer, but it is a risk factor. Women with LCIS have a 25 percent chance of developing breast cancer sometime within their lives.

The treatment options for LCIS range from close monitoring, with regular physical exams and annual mammograms, to bilateral prophylactic mastectomy—removal of both breasts—in women considered at extremely high risk. The use of tamoxifen, a hormonal form of therapy that blocks the growth of some breast cancer cells, is a new option being explored for treating LCIS. (See STAR trial on page 26.)

Ductal Carcinoma In Situ (DCIS)

Ductal carcinoma in situ, or DCIS, is a condition in which abnormal cells are found in the ducts of the breast. It is usually found by tiny specks of calcium, arranged in a particular pattern, on a mammogram. It is considered a pre-cancerous condition because these suspicious cells have not invaded the surrounding breast tissues. Over time, however, if left untreated, DCIS can become an invasive cancer.

Treatment for DCIS may range from localized surgery to remove only the abnormal area (lumpectomy) followed by radiation therapy, to total mastectomy for those women at extremely high risk. The decision is an individual one, and there is no consensus about the best treatment strategy for DCIS. Whatever *you* choose, it's the *right* decision.

Breast Cancer in Men

Breast cancer in men is rare, but it does occur. The most common symptoms include a lump in the breast or an abnormality in the nipple. If the cancer is detected at an early stage, survival is comparable to that of women. However, because most men are not aware that the disease can affect them, it is often detected at a more advanced stage.

Risk factors include having family members with breast cancer, especially with a genetic mutation, taking estrogen for a sex-change operation, and having higher estrogen levels due to liver diseases such as cirrhosis.

While the discussions throughout this book are generally geared toward women, most of the treatment options are equally applicable for men with breast cancer.

My Notes

"Schedule for My Check-Ups"
(and for my loved ones too!)

_____

_____

_____

_____

_____

_____

_____

_____

_____

_____

_____

_____

_____

_____

PART II:

Diagnosis and Treatment

A Diagnosis of Cancer.
What Does It Mean?

"I am so sorry to tell you that you have cancer." It is difficult to imagine more earth-shattering words. In an instant, your world turns upside down.

How can you possibly absorb such news? Some people express shock, others confusion. Some lash out and become angry, others withdraw and go into denial. Most are in a state of uncertainty and fear.

All of these reactions are totally normal. In fact, if you do not express one of these reactions, your physician may become worried about how you are coping.

That's the bad news. The good news is that there are very effective treatment options available today that will enable you to live a long and prosperous life. Yes, you will have some bumps in the road, but you can—*and will*—get over those.

From here on, it is very important that you try to understand everything you can about your diagnosis. What kind of cancer is it? At what stage was it caught? What treatment options are available? What side effects might result from those treatments?

Always remember that you are not alone! Whether it's your spouse or significant other, family members, close friends, and/or your healthcare team—at a time like this you will find how blessed you are to have these special people who will now embrace you. They will become an extraordinary source of comfort and support.

Keep in mind that cancer doesn't just strike *you*—it affects your loved ones as well. While it may be difficult to "let others do for you," it's very important for them to feel as though they can help you in your time of need. On the other hand, don't let them overpower you. Be strong. They need that from you, as they are hurting as well.

If you do not have anyone close to you, there are many support groups, community organizations, church programs, and other resources that can be of immense assistance. Contact them. Don't hesitate to ask for help and support. That is what they are there for—and they want to help. It will make them feel good that you called.

Understanding *Your* Breast Cancer

Most breast cancers are *invasive* breast cancers—cancerous cells that can invade nearby tissues, or enter the blood stream and lymphatic system, spreading to distant organs. (Non-invasive cancers are also called pre-cancers or cancer markers. Examples include LCIS and DCIS, which cannot spread, but simply indicate a significant risk of developing a cancer in the future.)

Invasive cancers are classified depending on their origin. The three most common are:

- *Infiltrating (or invasive) ductal carcinoma* (IDC), which begins in the ducts of the breast, is the most commonly diagnosed invasive breast cancer (80 percent).

- *Infiltrating (or invasive) lobular carcinoma* (ILC), which begins in the milk-producing glands of the breast, comprises approximately 15 percent of all invasive breast cancers.

- *Invasive mammary carcinoma* is a combination of the above.

In rare cases, breast cancer can begin in other areas of the breast. These include:

- *Inflammatory breast cancer* represents about 1 percent of all newly diagnosed breast cancers. Inflammatory breast cancer often makes the skin of the breast look red, feel warm, and develop an appearance similar to having an infection of the breast. The skin can resemble the outside of an orange (the so-called peau d'orange).

- *Tubular carcinoma* is a special type of cancer that accounts for about 2 percent of all invasive cancers. It is considered to be less aggressive than other forms of breast cancer.

- *Paget's disease* occurs in less than 1 percent of cases. It is characterized by eczema-like changes to the nipple (not the areola, which is the coloration around the nipple).

- *Phyllodes tumor* is a very rare type of tumor that forms in the connective tissues of the breast.

Stages of Breast Cancer

Once a breast cancer has been found, more tests will be done to see if the cancer has spread from the breast to other parts of the body, a process called *staging*. The following stages are used:

- **Stage 0:** The "cancer" is *in situ* without the ability to spread in its present state.

- **Stage I:** The cancer is confined to a single site in the breast. The tumor is small, less than 2 centimeters (3/4 inch) in size, and the cancer has not spread outside the breast. In this stage, the tumor is sometimes further classified as Stage IA (less than 0.5 cm) or Stage IB (0.5 cm - 1 cm).

- **Stage IIA:** The tumor is still less than 2 centimeters (3/4 inch) in size, but cancer has spread to involve your axillary (underarm) lymph nodes. Or, the tumor is larger, 2 - 5 centimeters (3/4 inch – 2 inches), but has not spread to your lymph nodes.

- **Stage IIB:** The tumor is larger than 5 centimeters (2 inches) in size but does not involve any lymph nodes. Or, the tumor is smaller but cancer has spread to involve your underarm lymph nodes.

- **Stage IIIA:** The tumor is smaller than 5 centimeters (2 inches) and the cancer has spread to the lymph nodes under your arm. The lymph nodes are attached to each other or to other structures. Or, the tumor is larger than 5 centimeters (2 inches) and the cancer has spread to the lymph nodes under the arm.

- **Stage IIIB:** The cancer has invaded the chest wall, skin or has spread to the internal mammary lymph nodes on the same side of the chest.

- **Stage IV:** The cancer has spread to distant locations in the body, which may include the bones, liver, lungs, brain or other faraway sites.

Family and Friends are Impacted Too

Unfortunately, you are not the only one impacted by the diagnosis of breast cancer. Your family and close friends are also affected. They have to deal with their own feelings as well as be sensitive to yours throughout treatment and recovery.

Often, family members absorb the brunt of a cancer patient's anger and frustration. They in turn may even lash back, expressing anger, hurt or frustration at their own powerlessness over the situation you are facing.

Remember that your family and close friends will be your most valuable source of support. They hopefully know when to simply listen, or when to encourage feelings to be shared. They can help make sure that the right questions are asked, or that questions are asked at all. And they can help you understand the incredible amount of new information now consuming your life.

This "second set of ears" can be extremely important. Studies have shown that the information retained by a patient after a cancer diagnosis is surprisingly incomplete. One study found that only 60 percent correctly recalled what their treatment entailed; 41 percent could not list even a single major treatment risk; and only 27 percent could name one treatment alternative.

Even when physicians are conscientious in communicating specific details regarding treatment and prognosis, patients often do not remember what was said. Hospital patients in general typically remember just over 50 percent of the information they receive from doctors about their diagnosis and treatment.

This figure drops to less than 25 percent for cancer patients. Distressing information may raise your anxiety level and significantly reduce your ability to remember details.

Hearing unexpected and unwanted information causes many people to focus on a particular word or sentence while the doctor keeps talking. **No problem.** Simply have it repeated. Or better yet, bring someone with you to all of your medical appointments and discuss with them the treatment options that have been presented.

It can be extremely helpful to bring a tape recorder so that you can listen in the privacy of your home to your doctor's explanation—over and over again, as many times as necessary. (Don't be surprised at how much you missed!)

Coping with cancer can be extremely challenging, but it doesn't have to be overwhelming—and it doesn't have to be undertaken alone.

Speak Up During Doctor Visits

Studies have shown that as many as three-quarters of the questions that cancer patients have are *not* asked during medical appointments. Why? Fear of humiliation in front of the doctor is the most commonly cited reason. Or you may worry that your doctor will misunderstand your motivation for questioning, or think that you are second-guessing his or her judgment. Of course, with so much going on, you don't want to ruin your relationship with your doctor.

Further, you may feel urgency about the amount of time you are taking from your doctor's "needier" patients. Feeling hurried obviously interferes with your ability to gather thoughts and clearly articulate questions.

Forget about hurting your doctor's feelings with questions, or taking up too much of his or her time. It is very important to keep in mind that *you're* the one with cancer. *You're* the one with the ultimate authority to make any treatment decisions. Your doctor is only a professional guide through *your* treatment and recovery.

That means *you* are ultimately responsible for adequately communicating to your doctor your concerns and needs, and any other treatments that you are considering. This is especially true with complementary and alternative therapies such as herbs, dietary supplements, megadoses of vitamins, and other measures.

About three-quarters of breast cancer patients use alternative therapies such as acupuncture, herbs, prayer or nutritional supplements, but only a third of these patients disclose their use of such treatments to their doctors. This lack of disclosure can sometimes lead to complications.

For example, some herbal supplements can skew the results of laboratory tests; some may increase the tendency to bleed during surgery; still others may cause side effects that are incorrectly attributed to an effective conventional treatment. **Talk to your doctor!**

Talking to Your Kids

What if you have young children? How do you tell *them* about your cancer? This is difficult enough with adult family members and friends, but it can be especially disconcerting with young children.

The reason for such difficulties is a fear of the questions the children may ask, particularly about the possibility of death. You may be concerned about causing too much anxiety and stress for your children, or you may think they will not understand. You want to protect them. That is a **totally normal** concern.

Such assumptions may make a difficult situation even worse for a child. Experts agree that communication is *essential* for children to be able to cope with the illness of a parent. So what should you tell the kids? And when?

Tell your children about your illness as soon as possible. Children as young as four and five *will* feel the tension in the home. When there's a delay, or if it's kept a family secret, they will build up resentment and quite possibly "imagine the worst."

But how to begin? The approach depends partly on each child's age and your personal relationship with them. Be as honest as possible, phrasing the discussion in terms of "love and hopefulness." Watch how they *individually* respond to what you are saying and continue your talk accordingly. Every child (and every adult, for that matter) will react and cope in their own unique way.

Reassure them that the cancer is not contagious and is not due to anything they did. (This is especially important for younger children.) Tell them that they will continue to be cared for no matter how family routines may temporarily be disrupted.

Even when the prognosis is poor, it is still possible to speak truthfully and with hope. For example: "Some people die from cancer, but many get better. I'm working very hard to be one of the people who gets better."

Along with providing honesty and reassurance to your children, watch for signs that they are not coping well. These can include significant changes in mood or personality, decreased appetite, withdrawal from friends and family, a sudden drop in grades, or behavior problems at school.

Second Opinions

Five words about second opinions—*"Don't hesitate to get one!"* If you feel at all uncomfortable with your doctor, if you consistently do not understand what is being recommended, or if you believe there are treatment options that are not being offered, you have the right—the obligation—to ask for a second opinion. Switch doctors if you feel the need.

Second opinions are often pursued for reasons far beyond the risk of misdiagnosis. Studies have shown that a woman's choice of a breast surgeon could be the most important factor in whether a small, early-stage breast cancer tumor is treated by lumpectomy or mastectomy—even when either procedure may be medically equivalent. Doctors sometimes perform procedures that they feel more comfortable with, rather than basing treatment decisions on the medical evidence available.

Even when there are no treatment alternatives to sort out, a second opinion can offer a fresh perspective. Maybe it can confirm a diagnosis or reinforce the wisdom of a course of treatment, and thus ease any doubts that you, or your family, may have. If you sense reluctance from your doctor about getting a second opinion, that may be all the more reason to get one. Remember, your physician works for *you.*

My Notes

"Questions to Ask My Doctor"
(To be answered DURING my appointment!)

_____

_____

_____

_____

_____

_____

_____

_____

_____

_____

_____

_____

_____

_____

Understanding Your Treatment Options

The primary treatment strategies for breast cancer have remained relatively consistent—surgery, radiation therapy, chemotherapy and hormonal therapy—and refinements in these techniques have made each of them *much* more effective. The relatively new option of monoclonal antibody therapy is also becoming available, as are a number of extremely promising new treatments now being evaluated in large-scale clinical trials.

While you will and should be given treatment options by your doctor, all of the final decisions will be left up to you. Keep this in mind—you can make no wrong decisions. Whatever option you might choose, at whatever stage of treatment, is the **right decision** for *you*.

Surgery

Some form of breast surgery will most likely be the initial treatment recommended. Surgery is a *local* treatment intended to remove the tumor and any surrounding tissue that might contain cancer cells. This differs from a *systemic*—system-wide—treatment such as chemotherapy, which attacks cancer cells throughout the body.

Surgery will also play a major role in staging the disease. Adequate sizing of the tumor once it's completely removed, and an analysis of the lymph nodes from the underarm, comprise the most important method of initial staging.

(If your tumor is relatively large at the time of diagnosis, your doctor may recommend an initial treatment of chemotherapy prior to surgery in an attempt to shrink the tumor, thus making the surgery more effective. This may also allow for the option of breast-conserving surgery to be considered.)

In general, there are two types of surgery available to treat breast cancer:

- *Lumpectomy plus axillary dissection*—This is breast-conserving surgery in which only the tumor is removed along with an extra margin of normal tissue. In addition, axillary (underarm) lymph nodes are sampled, usually through a separate incision. Lumpectomy/axillary dissection must be accompanied by radiation therapy for a period of 6-8 weeks. (Radiation therapy and its side effects are discussed later.)

- *Mastectomy*—This is surgery in which the entire breast and some lymph nodes are removed. The type of mastectomy most frequently performed for invasive cancers is called a *modified radical mastectomy*, which removes the breast and axillary contents but leaves the chest wall muscles intact. A *simple mastectomy*, which does not include an axillary lymph node dissection, may be performed for precancerous conditions (such as DCIS) or for prophylaxis (prevention).

The best surgical option for you depends on your individual situation. **Your choice is extremely important** and should be discussed at length with your surgeon. This may be the time to consider a second opinion, just to be sure that the surgical option you choose is indeed the most appropriate for you.

Lumpectomy

Lumpectomy, also referred to as breast-conservation surgery, involves removal of the breast lump with a surrounding margin of normal tissue to make sure that all of the cancer has been removed. Some lymph nodes will also be removed to be certain the cancer has not spread outside of the breast.

If examination of the removed tissue shows that cancer is present at its margin (the edge of the piece of removed tissue), the surgeon must then remove additional tissue. This second operation is called a *re-excision*. Even after a re-excision, in rare cases the margins may still be positive, necessitating an additional lumpectomy or even a "completion" mastectomy.

Lumpectomy is almost always followed by a course of radiation therapy to kill any cancer cells that might exist in any other portion of the breast but have not been detected. Rarely, in a very small (less than 0.5 cm) non-aggressive tumor, such as a tubular carcinoma, radiation may be avoided.

A disturbing number of studies have shown that many women who have had a lumpectomy for early-stage breast cancer are not receiving appropriate follow-up care, particularly radiation therapy after the surgery. *Radiation is an extremely important part of the treatment*; it greatly reduces the risk of local recurrence.

Lumpectomy (with axillary lymph node sampling) and radiation is a package deal. You cannot choose lumpectomy and then not follow through with radiation. Not having radiation greatly increases the risk of recurrence, something we definitely don't want and certainly can avoid.

Mastectomy

There are a number of "different" mastectomy procedures, although a modified radical mastectomy is clearly the most common.

In a *modified radical mastectomy*, the entire breast is removed as well as a number of axillary lymph nodes under the arm.

In a *simple* or *total mastectomy*, the surgeon removes only the breast, but does not remove lymph nodes from under the arm. This procedure is usually reserved for women with carcinoma in situ, where the cancer has clearly not invaded nearby tissues.

A more extensive procedure, a *radical mastectomy* (*Halsted radical mastectomy*) involves the removal of the breast tissue, chest muscles, and most of the lymph nodes in the underarm area. This type of surgery is rarely done today. If it is recommended, *definitely* get a second opinion.

Following a mastectomy, in the immediate post-operative period (within a week or two) you will be custom-fitted with a breast form called a *prosthesis*, which inserts into a special bra. When dressed, no one will be able to tell that you have had any surgery. In addition, there are an array of effective reconstructive procedures available to you. (We will discuss these shortly.)

Lumpectomy vs. Mastectomy

Perhaps the most difficult choice you will have to make in your treatment is deciding between lumpectomy and mastectomy when both options appear to be medically equivalent. Each has advantages and disadvantages. Both may be good options; again, there is **no wrong choice!**

The advantage in choosing lumpectomy is strictly cosmetic—you can preserve up to 90 percent of your breast. The disadvantage is that you must undergo radiation therapy and its potential side effects.

The advantage of mastectomy is that you don't need to have radiation, except in rare circumstances. The disadvantage, obviously, is the loss of your breast and the resulting cosmetic and psychological consequences.

What is the rate of success for lumpectomy vs. mastectomy? For Stage I and II cancers where lumpectomy is an option, the rates of long-term, disease-free survival appear to be identical. That's **good news!** With early cancer, either choice can be the correct choice.

What about the surgeries themselves? As it turns out, most of the problems are related to the axillary (underarm) part of the procedures. The risks of anesthesia, infection and bleeding are the same. The amount of pain and discomfort are nearly identical and—in fact—thankfully minimal. Most women require very few pain pills after either operation.

Both procedures take about an hour to perform and you should be invited to stay overnight in the hospital. They each may leave you with an area of numbness on the back of the arm. Both operations require that a drain (a plastic tube to drain off any liquids which may accumulate) be kept in place for 3 to 5 days.

Both lumpectomy and mastectomy have nearly the same incidence of arm swelling (lymphedema), which occurs in about 1 to 5 percent of cases. This may be slightly higher when you undergo lumpectomy and axillary lymph node dissection followed by radiation, but in no way should it dissuade you from choosing a lumpectomy, if that is your decision.

Following either procedure, you may want to use an electric razor for underarm shaving to minimize the risk of infection, as well as avoid using a deodorant on the side of the surgery. You will also be asked not to drive for a few days, unless absolutely necessary. However, within a few weeks you should be able to resume your normal activities, including routine shaving and deodorant use.

Side Effects of Surgery

Side effects that you may experience from your surgery will vary depending on the type of surgery involved as well as your own personal circumstances. Nausea and vomiting from anesthesia may be the most immediate side effects, especially for patients who have experienced these symptoms with anesthesia before. People who are susceptible to motion sickness, who have diabetes, or who are obese are also more prone to experience postoperative nausea and vomiting. Headaches, generalized body pains and fatigue are also very common and totally normal.

Nearly all patients are uncomfortable during the first few days following any surgery. Such discomfort can usually be controlled with minimal medication. Don't fear becoming addicted. Be pain-free and take your medications as prescribed. Don't wait until you develop severe pain before taking your pain relievers.

The Bottom Line

Most states mandate that you, the patient, must make the final decision regarding your surgery, and that you be provided with an "informed consent" form that lists your treatment options and their respective risks. We could not agree more. However, it has been shown in study after study that the majority of women (and their loved ones) ask the surgeon to make the final decision. That's okay, but remember that whatever your decision, there is no wrong choice. You and your surgeon should both be **comfortable** with your decision.

Sentinel Node Biopsy

In years past, when a woman underwent a lumpectomy or mastectomy, the surgeon would take out a large number of nearby lymph nodes to see if the cancer had spread. This could result in unwanted side effects, including some limitation of arm movement, pain, and often a condition known as *lymphedema,* in which fluid accumulates in the arm, causing pain and disfigurement.

Recently, researchers began theorizing that there might be a single lymph node—a "sentinel" node—that would be the first place to which cancer cells would spread. If that sentinel node could be identified, and if it was found to be free of cancer, then cancer may not have spread to the other lymph nodes. This might eliminate the need to do more extensive axillary lymph node dissections.

Recent techniques to identify the sentinel node (or nodes— sometimes there are two, three or even more), have proven to be accurate. Therefore, it is possible that a sentinel node biopsy will be recommended as part of your surgery. (Keep in mind, however, that your individual circumstances might necessitate the testing of additional lymph nodes, especially if your cancer was diagnosed at a more advanced stage.)

There are currently several methods that a surgeon might use to locate the sentinel node. One is to inject a blue dye near the breast tumor and track its path through the lymphatic system. The dye eventually accumulates in the sentinel node. Similarly, a small, safe amount of radioactive solution could be used, which likewise accumulates in the sentinel node. Most surgeons prefer to use a combination of these techniques.

While sentinel node biopsy is far from perfect, it appears to be an accurate measure for determining if the cancer has spread, saving many women from more extensive—and often unnecessary—surgery. Large-scale clinical trials are currently underway to verify the technique's effectiveness.

However, until the results of these trials adequately address the limitations of the technique (such as false-negative results and the potential for "under-staging" the disease, particularly in premenopausal women), the gold-standard remains at least an axillary lymph node sampling.

Radiation Therapy

Radiation therapy uses high energy x-rays directed at the location of the cancer cells. It is a *local* form of treatment used to destroy cancer cells that may remain after breast conservation surgery (lumpectomy). It may also be used for localized control of cancer cells that have spread to other parts of the body.

Prior to receiving radiation therapy, a process called a "simulation" will be undertaken by the radiation therapist. This involves identifying the specific areas to be targeted for radiation. This simulation may use x-rays, CT scans or other imaging studies to plan the direction of radiation. Small tattoo dots are placed on the area to be treated so that the subsequent radiation can be administered accurately and to the same area each time.

Radiation therapy is typically given 5 days a week for 6 to 8 weeks. Treatments last only minutes, although travel, waiting time, and talking with the medical staff can add up to an hour or so.

It is worth it. Radiation treatments for breast cancer play a *crucial* role in minimizing the risk of local recurrence (return) of the disease.

Side Effects of Radiation Therapy

The most common side effects of radiation therapy include sunburn-like changes to the skin, shriveling of the breast tissues, swelling with chronic pain, and injury to the organs in the path of the x-ray beams (ribs, lung and heart). Occasionally nausea occurs. In rare cases, radiation therapy causes a decrease in the number of blood cells in your body, resulting in anemia. Very rarely, radiation may result in the development of a secondary cancer, since radiation exposure, in and of itself, is a known carcinogen.

Fatigue is common during radiation therapy. Your body will use a lot of extra energy over the course of your treatment, and you may feel progressively more tired. Be sure to eat well, get plenty of rest, and sleep or nap as often as you feel the need.

It is common for the fatigue to last for 4 to 6 weeks after your treatment has been completed. Remember, your body has recently been severely traumatized. Surgery, anesthesia, radiation, and the psychological ordeal which you have been through may well have a cumulative impact.

The majority of skin reactions due to radiation therapy disappear a few weeks or months after the treatment has been completed. In some cases, the treated skin will remain slightly darker than it was before, and it may continue to be more sensitive to sun exposure.

During the course of radiation, wear loose, soft, cotton cloth-
ing over the treated area and protect it from the sun. When you wash,
use only lukewarm water and mild soap, then pat dry. Ask your doctor
or nurse to recommend skin care products that will help minimize
skin irritation.

Women who have a very small, early stage, non-aggressive
cancer, which has not spread to their lymph nodes, may want to weigh
the benefits of radiation therapy with the risks. However, for the vast
majority of women with breast cancer, radiation therapy remains an
extremely effective—and safe—treatment strategy.

Chemotherapy

Chemotherapy is the use of chemicals to kill cancer cells.
These chemicals are, unfortunately, poisons. Most chemotherapy drugs
are injected into veins; some are given by mouth. Chemotherapy is a
systemic (system-wide) treatment, meaning that the drugs flow through
the bloodstream to every part of the body to kill cancerous cells.

Chemotherapy is generally given in cycles; a treatment period is followed by a recovery period, then another treatment period,
and so on. This enables your body, particularly your blood cells, to
recover sufficiently for the next round of treatment.

Although a single chemotherapy drug can be used by itself,
most are given together (*combination chemotherapy*). Different chemotherapy drugs, with different actions, can often work together to
attack cancerous cells more effectively than a single drug acting alone.
Furthermore, combining different drugs can minimize the chance for
developing resistance to a particular drug. (See Appendix I for a listing of the most common chemotherapy drugs.)

Chemotherapy works by targeting reproducing and fast-grow-
ing cells throughout the body. This is a prime characteristic of cancer

cells, but it is unfortunately also a trait of certain normal cells. These include blood cells, the cells of the digestive tract, hair follicles, and others. (That is why certain chemotherapy drugs cause fatigue, nausea, temporary hair loss, etc.)

Therefore, each time chemotherapy is administered, it involves striking a balance between being strong enough to kill cancer cells, while, at the same time, minimizing injury to normal cells.

Side Effects of Chemotherapy

The most important side effect of chemotherapy is the lowering of your blood counts (immunosuppression). Because chemotherapy can reduce the normal functioning of the bone marrow, where most blood cells are produced, it can cause:

- Anemia – you may have less energy.
- Low platelets – you may bruise or bleed easily.
- Low antibodies – you may be more susceptible to infections.

Fatigue is a common side effect of chemotherapy. It can range from feeling "blah" to "total exhaustion." Some of the things you can do to minimize fatigue during your treatment include getting enough rest, eating a well-balanced diet, and limiting your activities. Do only the things that are important to you—and don't hesitate to ask for help!

Feeling nauseous is common during chemotherapy. Your doctor can prescribe anti-nausea medication to help. But there are also some things that you can do yourself, including eating small, frequent meals and eating only those foods you desire, even if they are "unusual." (See Appendix II for a listing of the most common anti-nause medications.)

You will also be more prone to infections during treatment. **Eat healthy** and **get plenty of rest.** Avoid large crowds or individuals who have a cold, infection, or any contagious disease. (Not that we shouldn't anyway.)

In most cases, chemotherapy can damage your ovaries, causing them to stop producing estrogen and resulting in instant menopause. If you are still in your child-bearing years and are considering having more children, it is important to talk with your physician prior to chemotherapy. Studies indicate that previous chemotherapy treatment does not have an impact on later pregnancies, but a waiting period may be wise.

Hot flashes, vaginal dryness, or painful intercourse can also occur as estrogen production is reduced by chemotherapy. Your doctor can prescribe treatments, including a number of medications, dietary changes and vaginal lubricants, which can help alleviate such nagging symptoms and unwanted changes in your lifestyle.

Hair loss commonly occurs with chemotherapy. It doesn't happen to all women, but when it does, it is one of the most obvious side effects. For many women, this is one of the most difficult parts of treatment. It is the ultimate insult. But, your hair *will* grow back—and it often comes back looking better than it did before! In the interim, there are many cosmetics, apparel options and wigs that can help you look beautiful and feel better about yourself.

Hormonal Therapy

Some types of breast cancer are stimulated by naturally occurring hormones such as estrogen. Hormonal therapy targets cancers that are fed by your own hormones. Like chemotherapy, hormonal therapy is a systemic—system-wide—therapy, which means that it affects cells throughout the body.

If tests show that your breast cancer is responsive to your natural hormones, it will be described as *estrogen receptor-positive* or *progesterone receptor-positive*. This means that any remaining cancer cells may continue to grow when these hormones are present in your body. Hormonal therapy may therefore be used to block the body's natural hormones from fueling these cancer cells.

Tamoxifen (Nolvadex®) is the most widely used form of hormonal therapy. It has been available for over two decades to treat patients with advanced stage breast cancer. It is currently being used as additional treatment for *early* stage disease. New studies indicate that taking tamoxifen not only acts as a *preventive* measure to minimize the risk of cancer coming back (recurring), but it also provides a protective effect against developing cancer in the opposite breast.

Tamoxifen works by interfering with the activity of estrogen, which has been shown to promote the growth of cancer cells that are estrogen-receptor positive. Another hormonal drug, raloxifene (Evista®), previously used as a treatment for osteoporosis, has been shown to act in a manner very similar to tamoxifen.

The potential benefits of both tamoxifen and raloxifene for reducing the incidence of breast cancer are so significant that the National Cancer Institute has begun the STAR trial—the Study of Tamoxifen and Raloxifene—to see just how well these drugs perform and to see if one is better than the other. Preliminary results from this trial are expected within the next few years. (See STAR trial on page 26.)

<u>Side Effects of Hormonal Therapy</u>

There are risks associated with both tamoxifen and raloxifene. Side effects of tamoxifen include hot flashes, nausea, vaginal spotting (small amounts of blood), or decreased fertility in younger women. In addition, tamoxifen has been associated with an increased risk of uterine cancer, as well as blood clots forming in the legs. Some of these clots may travel to the lungs, resulting in a condition known as a pulmonary embolism. Less common side effects include depression, vaginal itching, bleeding or discharge, loss of appetite, cataracts, headache, acne and weight gain.

Furthermore, recent studies appear to indicate that tamoxifen only has a beneficial impact for up to five years. After that, tamoxifen may have an opposite, estrogen-*promoting* effect. We still don't know why.

Although the side effects of raloxifene are less well known, the aggravation of menopausal symptoms appears to be significant. Currently, there does not seem to be an increase in the incidence of uterine cancer with raloxifene. Comparable studies on the time-span benefit for raloxifene are not yet available.

(Refer to Tables I and II for a summary of treatment options and their respective risks and benefits.)

Monoclonal Antibody Therapy
(Immunotherapy)

Monoclonal antibody therapy uses compounds called antibodics, which are proteins made by the body's immune system to fight foreign and infectious agents. Monoclonal antibody therapy is often referred to as immunotherapy or biological therapy.

With this kind of therapy, researchers are trying to entice substances in the immune system called "monoclonal antibodies" to latch onto specific sites on the surface of cancer cells—killing them in the process, while leaving untouched those cells that do not have such a cancer marker.

The first such monoclonal antibody to be developed as a treatment for breast cancer was a drug called trastuzumab, more commonly known by its brand name, Herceptin® (Genentech). Specifically, herceptin targets cancer cells that have an abundance of sites called *HER2-neu* oncogenes on their cell surface. When many of these sites are present ("overexpressed"), it is easier for herceptin to find targets to latch onto. It then inhibits the cancer cells' ability to grow and proliferate.

Table I:
Treatment Options for Invasive Breast Cancer Risks and Benefits

Treatment	Risks	Benefits	Comments
Surgery: Lumpectomy/axillary dissection	Radiation	Breast preservation	Both procedures limit your arm motion for 3-7 days. Some patients have long-term reduction in arm motion. Arm swelling (lymphedema) may occur.
Modified Radical Mastectomy	Cosmetic deformity	Avoidance of radiation side effects.	
Radiation	Sunburn, changes in breast consistency, chronic pain in breast or arm, fatigue, nausea, injury to lungs, ribs, heart.	Preserves 75-90% of own breast tissue, avoiding the need for reconstruction.	The chances associated with these side effects vary greatly. Some patients experience none of them. Treatment takes place 5 days/week for 6-8 weeks.
Chemotherapy	Nausea/vomiting, hair loss, immuno-suppression (increased risk of infection), fatigue.	Treats distant disease, decreases recurrence risk.	The need for chemotherapy depends on many factors that may not be known at the initial consultation (e.g., lymph node involvement, estrogen/progesterone receptors, HER2-neu oncogene status).
Hormonal Therapy (Tamoxifen)	Increases risk for uterine cancer, blood clots, menopausal symptoms (hot flashes), cataracts, hypertension, headaches.	Decreases recurrence rates by up to 30-35%. Protects the opposite breast from developing cancer by 35-40%.	Current recommended treatment is for a five-year period. May be of limited benefit thereafter.

Table II:
Treatment Options for Ductal Carcinoma in Situ
Risks and Benefits

Treatment	Risks	Benefits	Comments
Surgery: Lumpectomy	Radiation	Breast preservation	
Simple Mastectomy	Cosmetic deformity	Avoidance of radiation side effects.	Simple mastectomy may limit your arm motion for 3-7 days.
Radiation	Sunburn, changes in breast consistency, chronic pain in breast or arm, fatigue, nausea, injury to lungs, ribs, heart.	Preserves 75-90% of own breast tissue, avoiding the need for reconstruction.	The chances associated with these side effects vary greatly. Some patients experience none of them. Treatment takes place 5 days/week for 6-8 weeks.
Chemotherapy	Not indicated in the treatment of DCIS.		
Hormonal Therapy (Tamoxifen)	Increases risk for uterine cancer, blood clots, menopausal symptoms (hot flashes), cataracts, hypertension, headaches.	May offer protection from the development of invasive cancer on the opposite side.	Current recommended treatment is for a five-year period. May be of limited benefit thereafter.

Studies have shown that an overexpression of the HER2-neu oncogene occurs in at least one-third of all women with breast cancer. Therefore, developing monoclonal antibodies such as herceptin that specifically attack the HER2-neu oncogene has become an extremely important area of breast cancer research. Unfortunately, while a third of women with breast cancer may potentially benefit from herceptin, a much smaller percentage will show a significant positive response.

Cancerous tissue is usually tested for overexpression of the HER2-neu oncogene. Pathology labs keep tissues for a number of years, so if your tissue was not previously tested for HER2-neu, you can still request that this be done.

Side Effects of Immunotherapy

A small percentage of patients who take herceptin develop allergic reactions to the drug. In rare cases, these have been fatal (although some of these deaths may have been the result of other complications from the patients' cancers.) Most patients experience pain at the site of injection. Herceptin should not be used in conjunction with other drugs that may injure or weaken the heart (such as Adriamycin®). Nonetheless, herceptin is considered to be one of the least toxic breast cancer drugs currently available.

Breast Reconstruction

Reconstructive surgery following mastectomy does not treat cancer, but only attempts to restore a natural appearance. It is important to realize that a reconstructed breast will look and feel different; it will never be like your own breast, nor will it exactly match the remaining one. Nonetheless, recent advances in techniques have been remarkable.

The breast may be reconstructed with implants or with tissue from other parts of the body:

- *Implants* - There are two types of implants: saline (salt water) and silicone (liquid plastic), although the use of silicone implants has been dramatically reduced. The implants are generally placed under the chest wall muscle. A tissue expander—an inflatable implant containing a valve for saline injection—is used to stretch the tissues. When the appropriate size is achieved, the tissue expander is replaced with a permanent implant.

- *Tissue Flaps* - Muscle, blood vessels, fat and skin from another part of the body can be used to form a new breast. Often this involves taking tissue from the lower stomach area (TRAM flap), back or buttocks.

The TRAM flap is the most commonly used procedure when reconstruction with your own tissues is chosen. It is a lengthy procedure (3-4 hours of surgery) requiring careful consideration. It definitely is not for everyone. Discuss it thoroughly with your surgeon.

Additional smaller surgeries are often needed to complete the reconstructive process. These may involve creating and tattooing the nipple, and making changes to the opposite breast (with a reduction or perhaps a lift) to help create symmetry.

Complications of Breast Reconstruction

Breast implants can pose some difficulty in future breast imaging. Both saline-filled and silicone gel-filled implants are opaque to x-rays, meaning that any breast tissue behind the implant may not be seen on a mammogram. If you have breast implants, be sure to tell the mammography technician so that special "displacement" views can be taken. Remember, *it is still important to have regular mammograms!*

Although some people believe that silicone gel implants can cause debilitating illnesses, especially autoimmune diseases, there is no current evidence to support such conclusions. Breast implants, especially for cancer patients, have become much safer. Your surgeon should take the time to discuss implant options with you.

Breast implants may result in chronic pain due to scar formation. In addition, they may migrate up or down the chest, requiring replacement. Rarely, over time, they may leak, resulting in shrinkage and again requiring replacement.

Finally, keep in mind that there are no time limits to choosing reconstruction. If you decline breast reconstruction now, you can still consider it later, even years down the line.

New Treatments on the Horizon

Many new treatment options will soon be emerging from ongoing clinical trials. For example, *gene therapy* is a treatment that modifies genes and then reinjects them into your body to fight cancer. With gene therapy, researchers are trying to stimulate the body's natural abilities to fight the disease more effectively, or to make the cancer more sensitive to other cancer-fighting treatments.

Another avenue of research is focusing on attacking the *blood vessels* of a tumor rather than the tumor itself. The process by which new blood vessels are formed is called angiogenesis. Such new cancer-fighting strategies involve the development of *angiogenesis inhibitors*—compounds that act to interrupt this process of tumor blood vessel formation. When tumors are deprived of their blood supply, they starve and go away.

Researchers are also focusing on a new class of drugs that inhibit the production of estrogen in a fashion similar to tamoxifen. These so-called *aromatase inhibitors* target a specific enzyme (the aromatase enzyme) that plays a key role in the production of estrogen in postmenopausal women.

There are many other promising avenues of research. If your disease is in a more advanced stage, we urge you to consider enrolling in a clinical trial to test one of these potentially revolutionary new treatment options. Ask your doctor if there are any clinical trials that may be appropriate for you.

Complementary and Alternative Therapies

Cancer patients are turning to so-called "complementary and alternative therapies" in extraordinary numbers. While some refer to such treatments as "complementary," and others as "alternative," and still others as "complementary *and* alternative," there actually is a difference.

A therapy is generally called "complementary" when it is used *in addition to* conventional treatments. *Complementary* therapies are not intended to cure disease, but rather to help control symptoms and improve well-being. For example, a patient may practice meditation to reduce stress, or undergo acupuncture treatments to alleviate chronic pain. Other examples of complementary therapies include massage, yoga and aromatherapy, among others.

Alternative therapies refer to treatments that are intended to be used *instead of* conventional treatments. They are sometimes promoted as "cancer cures." Some alternative therapies, especially if taken in large doses, can counteract the benefits of standard medicines and skew lab test results. Examples of alternative therapies include megadoses of a particular vitamin or mineral, shark cartilage, and other such products. Many are expensive, some are harmful, and none are proven.

Some doctors are concerned that the use of non-traditional treatments may lead patients to abandon standard medical care. However, it appears that many cancer patients view the use of complementary therapies as a way in which they can **take control** of their situation and become more personally involved in promoting a healthy recovery.

It is estimated that up to 75 percent of breast cancer patients are combining traditional medical treatments with complementary or alternative therapies. But *only a third* discuss their use of such therapies with their doctor.

Most complementary therapies, and many alternative thera-

81

pies, are perfectly safe if used appropriately—and not at the expense of traditional medical treatment. You can only know for sure, however, if you talk with your doctor.

In addition, we can't caution you enough about treatments or therapies that promise you all, deliver nothing, and deplete your finances in the process! Don't allow yourself to get fooled. It could cost you more than money—it could cost your health.

Clinical Trials

Most successful treatments used today began as clinical trials, which are studies designed to evaluate the safety and effectiveness of a new treatment. Those patients who participate in such trials are the first to potentially benefit from any improved therapies. Clinical trials take place in many hospitals across the country and typically involve three *phases*:

- **Phase I** – This is the first time that a new drug or treatment is tested in people. It usually involves only a small number of patients, but gives an early indication of the drug's safety and potential effectiveness. Side effects, while unpredictable, are carefully monitored.

- **Phase II** – A phase II trial continues to test the safety of a drug, and attempts to measure how well it will actually work. A larger number of patients are enrolled in phase II trials so physicians can better assess the anti-cancer impact of the treatment. Side effects continue to be monitored.

- **Phase III** – By this time, the new drug or treatment has shown early promise in treating a particular disease. The treatment will now be compared to a current standard. A participant will be randomly assigned to receive either the new treatment or a standard treatment (the "control group"). Phase III trials enroll large numbers of people and are conducted at medical centers nationwide.

All clinical trial participants receive the best care possible, and their reactions to all treatments are closely monitored. If the treatment does not seem to be helping, your doctor will remove you from the study. In addition, *you* may choose to leave the trial at any time. If you leave a study for any reason, standard care and treatment are still provided. There is <u>no</u> penalty for leaving a clinical trial.

Unfortunately, participation rates in clinical trials by eligible breast cancer patients—especially older and minority patients—are extremely low. This has major implications for advances in breast cancer treatment.

Nearly all of the treatment options that are available to you today have come from previous breast cancer clinical trials. These include modern mammographic screening techniques; the use of adjuvant chemotherapy and hormonal therapies; and the combination of radiation therapy with lumpectomy for the effective treatment of breast cancer.

A common misunderstanding about contemporary clinical trials is the belief that you will receive no treatment if you are enrolled as a "control" group. Nothing could be further from the truth. In fact, if enrolled, you are guaranteed to receive, at the very least, the currently available treatment option. No "sugar pills!" In addition, enrollment in clinical trials brings you "under the microscope." You may be observed, screened, tested and monitored far more carefully than someone who has chosen not to participate.

If you believe you are eligible for a clinical trial, or would simply like to know more about them, ask your doctor. You can also call the National Cancer Institute's Cancer Information Service at 1-800-4CANCER for more information.

A Few Words About Pain

Not all cancer patients experience pain. Yet when pain does occur, it can often be treated effectively with prescription or nonprescription pain relievers. Even complementary approaches such as re-laxation techniques and herbs can be used with good results.

Far too often, cancer pain is *not* adequately treated, and this can generate side effects of its own: headaches, weakness, sleepless-ness, loss of appetite, anxiety, depression, and feelings of helpless-ness.

Sometimes, pain is associated with your treatment, such as discomfort following surgery or skin irritation from radiation. This type of pain usually decreases over time, and medications are avail-able to alleviate it during the course of treatment.

Pain can also be associated with the cancer itself. This can arise from a tumor causing pressure on adjacent organs, nerves or bones, or a cancer-related blockage of a particular blood vessel. When cancer metastasizes (spreads) to other organs, it can cause direct pain in those sites as well.

It is not always possible to identify or treat a single source of pain. In such cases, there are a number of pain-relief options. Medi-cines that relieve pain are called analgesics. Analgesics act on the nervous system to provide temporary relief for pain. Nonprescription pain relievers, sometimes called "over-the-counter" pain remedies, include aspirin, acetaminophen and ibuprofen.

For more severe pain, prescription pain relievers, in particu-lar opioid narcotics, may be prescribed. These include: codeine, hydrocodone, hydromorphone, levorphanol, meperidine, methadone and morphine, among others. Also, a transdermal (through the skin) fentanyl patch may be used for chronic pain.

Sometimes pain can be relieved without the use of non-prescription or prescription medicines. Such treatments include acupuncture, relaxation techniques, herbal supplements, and visual-ization/imagery.

Don't wait until you are experiencing significant pain to take your medication. Pain is much easier to control when it is mild rather than severe. You should take your pain medicine regularly and as often as your doctor recommends, or as often as you feel the need. While you may feel concerned about developing an addiction—forget it. You won't. **Be comfortable.** Don't hurt.

PART III:

Recovery

Recovery

Thanks to the many advances in breast cancer treatment, especially in the past decade, more women are not only surviving breast cancer, but are living healthy, disease-free lives long after treatment.

You are now a "breast cancer survivor." **GREAT! You've recovered!** You will finally get your life back to normal.

However, as such, you will face a unique set of physical and emotional issues in the process. For example, if you wish to have children, you may be concerned about the timing of pregnancy with respect to treatment, or whether your treatment will have affected your ability to get pregnant at all. You may also be concerned about premature menopause, or the advisability of hormone replacement therapy.

Also, regardless of age, the fear of recurrence will always (to some extent) be present. Don't let it take over your life!

Adequate nutrition and exercise will have a tremendous impact on your recovery—not to mention your overall health and well-being. Good nutrition is *absolutely essential,* but it is not always easy to maintain. For example, various treatments can suppress your appetite, as can anxiety and stress.

In general, if appetite becomes a concern, you may want to plan meals and snacks that include your favorite foods. Preparing more frequent, smaller meals may be helpful. Talk with your doctor or a nutritionist about a meal plan that meets your needs.

Exercise, even on a minimal scale, has been shown to have a profound impact on recovery in cancer patients—not only in terms of physical recuperation but also for emotional well-being.

While your strength and stamina may vary at different times during your treatment and recovery, you will still be able to perform some type of moderate exercise. Remember, it can be tailored to your individual needs.

Emotional Issues

Let's step aside from physical issues for a moment. The nagging fear of cancer returning can have an *emotional* impact on your health.

Anxiety, sadness and temporary depression can understandably accompany your diagnosis and treatment; these will subside with time. In the interim, there are medications available that can help, not to mention complementary therapies such as meditation and relaxation techniques.

Ongoing depression is more serious and can have a profound impact on your quality of life. It is therefore important to talk to your doctor if you suffer from extended bouts of anxiety, sadness, or significant changes in lifestyle which just aren't "you." Depression *can* be treated, but you must let your doctor know. Don't be embarrassed. **You are not alone.** In fact, your doctor will worry about you if you *don't* complain about feeling sad or depressed at some point.

Don't conceal your feelings and concerns, especially from family, close friends and your healthcare team. There will be times during your treatment and recovery when everything might seem to be just too much to handle. That's normal, that's expected, and that's the time to reach for help. Don't deal with such feelings alone.

Fatigue and exhaustion can also have a direct impact on your emotional well-being. If you are refreshed and alert, you can handle more. So get plenty of rest, pace yourself, and make time for all of the activities that you enjoy!

Intimacy and Sexuality

Sexuality fulfills a significant need for closeness, and there is no reason that it cannot continue during your treatment and recovery. Yet some pervasive myths regarding sexuality and cancer still abound. Sex will *not* make your cancer worse and it *won't* cause a recurrence. In fact, the intimacy from sexual activity actually provides important emotional benefits throughout your recovery process.

Sexual activity is safe during treatment. There may be times when sex may be temporarily painful, or when a period of rest and recuperation from *all* activities may be called for. But in general, if you're in the mood, enjoy it!

Be open and honest with your partner; hopefully your partner will be open and honest with you as well. Periods of time may pass where your desire for intimacy is subdued, followed by periods involving an intense need for intimacy. A little patience, a lot of communication, and an abundance of love can be especially important at this time in your life.

Financial Issues

Beyond its physical and emotional tolls, cancer can be a difficult financial challenge as well. You may have been working full-time when you were diagnosed and may need to take an extended leave of absence. In addition, your spouse and other family members may have to take time off from their work to help you.

Studies have shown that families can spend a significant proportion of their income on cancer care. Often it is necessary to take out a loan or second mortgage, spend savings, or get a second job to finance treatment. This clearly adds additional stress to an already difficult situation.

Don't be embarrassed about any financial difficulties you might be having. Without question, everyone—including most creditors—will understand. (This is *cancer*, not an overextended credit card.) Ask your doctor to refer you to a social worker who can recommend financial assistance programs. You may also be able to obtain assistance directly from the hospital, or from community organizations such as your church. *Ask!*

Consider talking to a financial advisor. A good one can negotiate extended payment plans, help you prioritize expenses, and perhaps suggest the most effective way to use your assets. You may also want to consider a program offered by the American Cancer Society called "Taking Charge of Money Matters," which includes workshops on many financial issues facing families with cancer. You can call them at 1-800-227-2345 for more information.

Cancer and Your Career

If you were working before your cancer diagnosis, count on returning to your job. You will appreciate it all the more!

When you return to work, you may find that some people simply aren't sure how to react. They may be scared, worried, or just don't understand what you are dealing with. Unfortunately, outdated notions still persist about cancer, especially if the disease has not directly touched a person's family.

In the beginning, you may have to take some time to simply talk with your co-workers about your illness and recovery. If you need help, ask your manager or someone in the Human Resources department for assistance. If you work for a large company, there will be other employees who are cancer survivors. Consider forming a workplace cancer support group to discuss cancer- and job-related issues.

It is estimated that 80 percent of people with cancer return to work after their diagnosis. Yet 1 in 4 cancer survivors will experience some form of employment discrimination. If you feel that you are being treated unfairly, don't hesitate to take additional actions within or outside of the company.

Changing Jobs

If you are looking for a new job after your cancer treatment ends, it is important to anticipate that your cancer history may become an issue. Keep in mind that you have just overcome one of the biggest challenges you could possibly face. Take that **confidence** into the job interview! Here are some additional suggestions from the National Cancer Institute:

- Don't discriminate against yourself. Look at your current skills and capabilities and apply for jobs you know you can do, and do well—perhaps better than anyone else.

- Organize your resume to your best advantage. For example, a chronological resume should avoid questions raised by your treatment or recovery. Avoid gaps, possibly by organizing your resume by skills or achievements instead of by dates of employment.

- Get a letter from your doctor (on office or hospital stationery) that explains your health situation to potential employers. Have the doctor specifically address your physical ability to perform the type of work you are seeking and to confirm that you are now in good health.

- Be honest about your cancer history if an employer or an application asks.

- Qualify your "yes" with **positive** statements about your current health.

- Don't volunteer health information if not asked. You have no legal responsibility to mention your cancer unless it directly relates to the job you seek. Information needs to be divulged on a "need-to-know" basis.

- Avoid sounding defensive. Be confident!

Personal Support

You may be fortunate enough to have family members and close personal friends help you during treatment and recovery. Keep in mind that your cancer is affecting *them* as well—physically through fatigue from caregiving responsibilities, and emotionally with their understandable anxiety about your illness. Whatever emotions you are experiencing, chances are they are feeling many of the same.

Cancer causes great upheavals in the way family members interact, with traditional roles sometimes turned upside down and inside out. Parents might look to their children for emotional support at a time when the children themselves need it most. Teenagers might have to assume major household responsibilities. Young children can revert to infantile behavior as a way of dealing with their frustrations.

Patience, understanding, and examining what's truly important can often help families get through these times—and be much stronger and closer as a result. Relax housekeeping standards, or have everyone pitch in to prepare meals. (It can be a lot of fun!) Children can, and often do, take on more household chores than they have handled before.

You will also have an ongoing need for support from your healthcare team. This includes having a *two-way* dialogue with your doctor about any concerns that you have. As we mentioned before, take full advantage of your doctor's time during office visits:

- When going to meet your doctor or nurse, bring someone with you. It helps to have another person listen to what is being said and to think of questions to ask during the consultation.
- Write out your questions beforehand; don't forget to discuss any issue.
- Write down or record the answers you get, and make sure you understand what you are hearing.
- Ask your questions. If you feel you are not receiving adequate answers to your concerns, ask where you can find them.

Support Groups

Is a support group for you? Cancer support groups are designed to provide a confidential atmosphere where you can talk frankly about the challenges that you are facing with others in a similar situation. Participants gather to exchange information, discuss practical problems (such as managing side effects), or simply to lend emotional support.

Your healthcare staff should be able to provide you with specific information about local support groups. Some meet informally with just survivors; others are directed by healthcare professionals. Take the time to find a support group that makes you feel comfortable and fits with your specific needs. If you don't feel you want to be part of a support group, that's **perfectly all right** too.

Many survivors, however, are surprised at how important their support group meetings become. There's nothing quite like sharing a concern or experience with someone who knows—on the most personal of levels—exactly what you're going through.

Coping With Recurrence

The news that the cancer has come back—recurred—is a time for understandable anxiety and fear. But it should *not* be a time for panic.

New advances in surgical techniques, radiation, chemotherapy and other treatments are constantly becoming available. On the immediate horizon are potentially *revolutionary* advances in cancer treatment, especially with our rapidly unfolding knowledge about the human genetic code.

At a time such as this, don't be afraid to show your emotions. Shock, grief and despair are normal—and understandable. Gather your family and friends around you. They have been invaluable since you were first diagnosed, and they will most certainly be supportive now.

Reassess your healthcare team if you feel the need. Make sure you are comfortable with your doctor and staff. Are they compassionate? Are they willing to consider a broad range of new treatment options? Are you satisfied with the care that you have received to date? If not, don't hesitate to get a referral, or a second opinion, if you are considering new treatment options.

Most important of all—*don't give up!* Consider this as another bump in the road, although a rather difficult one. There are many, many women living well and disease-free today who have had recurrences of their own a long time ago. There is no reason why you can't be one of them!

Living With Advanced Disease

If your disease should become advanced, simple day-to-day activities that you once enjoyed may at times be more difficult, occasionally even overwhelming. There will be good days and bad days.

Keep in mind that the reality of your advanced disease must *always* be balanced with the **hope** that one of the remarkable new treatments now emerging from clinical trials will be the perfect treatment developed just for *you*. Never give up hope.

Be responsible, however, especially in terms of your loved ones. Update your will, prepare a Durable Power of Attorney for Health Care, and attend to any other matters of personal importance. Quite frankly, these are things that all of us should address long before illness ever becomes an issue.

Some people find cancer is a spur to do the fun, adventurous things they've always wanted to do but have simply put off. Go for it! Pursue travel plans, take on hobbies that have always interested you, or simply take the time to "catch your breath." Cancer and its treatment can be intensive, frustrating, exhausting, and often overwhelming. Step back and enjoy what truly makes you happy. Live life to the fullest!

My Notes

"A To-Do List for Life"
(Things that truly bring me happiness!)

_____

_____

_____

_____

_____

_____

_____

_____

_____

_____

_____

Appendices

Appendices I & II

Common Breast Cancer Drugs
Common Anti-Nausea Medications

Appendix I

Common Breast Cancer Drugs *

Drug (Trade Name) Manufacturer	Indications	Possible Side Effects	Method of Administration
Anastrozole (Arimidex®) AstraZeneca Pharmaceuticals	For advanced, estrogen-positive breast cancer in postmenopausal women whose disease has progressed following tamoxifen therapy.	Flushing, mild nausea, vomiting, increased bone and tumor pain, hot flashes.	Oral (tablet)
Bleomycin (Blenoxane®) Bristol-Myers Squibb	For palliative treatment of breast cancer.	Mild fever, chills, stomatitis, anorexia, skin changes, hyper-sensitivity, hair loss, lung fibrosis.	Injection (IV)
Capecitabine (Xeloda®) Roche Oncology	For advanced breast cancer that is resistant to paclitaxel and has not responded to anthracycline-containing chemotherapy.	Fatigue, fever, diarrhea, nausea, vomiting, stomatitis, anorexia, abdominal pain, constipation, skin irritation.	Oral (tablet)

Common Breast Cancer Drugs

Drug (Trade Name) Manufacturer	Indications	Possible Side Effects	Method of Administration
Cyclophosphamide (Cytoxan®) Bristol-Myers Squibb	For the primary treatment of breast cancer.	Hair loss, heart failure, nausea vomiting, anorexia, diarrhea, stomatitis, cystitis.	Oral (tablet), Injection (IV)
Dexrazoxane (Zinecard®) Pharmacia Oncology	Used to lessen the risk of heart damage that might result from certain cancer medicines.	Pain at injection site.	Injection (IV)
Docetaxel (Taxotere®) Aventis Pharmaceutical	For advanced breast cancer that has progressed following primary chemotherapy.	Allergic reactions, fluid retention, inflammation, heart failure, fever, chills, hair loss, skin and nail changes.	Injection (IV)
Doxorubicin (Adriamycin®) Pharmacia Oncology	For the primary treatment of breast cancer.	Mouth sores, irregular heartbeat, pain at injection site, heart failure, nausea, hair loss.	Injection (IV)
Doxorubicin-Liposomal (Doxil®) ALZA	For the primary treatment of breast cancer.	Inflammation, heart failure, fever, nausea, skin reaction.	Injection (IV)
Epirubicin (Ellence®) Pharmacia Oncology	For the primary treatment of breast cancer.	Bleeding, mouth sores, fever, chills, nausea, heart failure, hair loss.	Injection (IV)

Drug (Trade Name) Manufacturer	Indications	Possible Side Effects	Method of Administration
Epoitin Alfa (Procrit®) Ortho-Biotech	For the treatment of anemia associated with chemotherapy or radiation.	Headaches, joint and bone pain, nausea.	Injection (IV), or subcutaneous injection
Exemestane (Aromasin®) Pharmacia Oncology	For advanced, estrogen-positive breast cancer in postmenopausal women whose disease has progressed following tamoxifen therapy.	Cough, hoarseness, fever, chills, increased blood pressure, back or side pain, depression, swelling, hot flashes, fatigue.	Oral (tablet)
Filgrastim (Neupogen®) Amgen	For the treatment of anemia, specifically the decrease in white blood cells associated with chemotherapy or radiation.	Nausea, vomiting, bone pain, hair loss, diarrhea.	Injection (IV), or subcutaneous injection.
Fluorouracil or 5-FU (Adrucil®) Roche Oncology	For the primary treatment of breast cancer.	Diarrhea, hearburn, stomatitis, nausea, vomiting, dermatitis, inflammation of the vein, skin reaction.	Injection (IV)
Gemcitabine (Gemzar®) Eli Lilly	For advanced breast cancer that is resistant to paclitaxel and has not responded to anthracycline-containing chemotherapy.	Shortness of breath, stomatitis, swelling, nausea, inflammation of the vein.	Injection (IV)

Drug (Trade Name) Manufacturer	Indications	Possible Side Effects	Method of Administration
Goserelin (Zoladex®) Astra Zeneca	For the treatment of estrogen-positive breast cancer.	Irregular heartbeat, heart failure, nausea, hot flashes, pain on implant.	Implanted under the skin.
Letrozole (Femara®) Novartis	For advanced, estrogen-positive breast cancer in postmenopausal women as a first-line treatment or whose disease has progressed following anti-estrogen therapy.	Shortness of breath, blood clots, nausea, headaches, hot flashes.	Oral (tablet)
Megestrol (Megace®) Bristol-Myers Squibb	Palliative treatment of breast cancer.	Bleeding, changes in menstrual flow, anorexia, edema, hot flashes, weight gain.	Oral (suspension and tablet)
Mitomycin (Mutamycin®) Bristol-Myers Squibb	For the treatment of advanced breast cancer.	Nausea, vomiting, stomatitis, liver failure, diarrhea, fever.	Injection (IV)
Mitoxantrone (Novantrone®) Immunex	Palliative treatment of breast cancer.	Seizures, heart/kidney failure, stomatitis, hair loss.	Injection (IV)
Paclitaxel (Taxol®) Bristol-Myers Squibb	For the treatment of node-positive breast cancer in conjunction with standard doxorubicin-containing combination chemotherapy.	Myalgia, liver failure, hair loss, irregular heartbeat, hyper-sensitivity, peripheral neuropathy, fever, electrolyte abnormalities.	Injection (IV)

Drug (Trade Name) Manufacturer	Indications	Possible Side Effects	Method of Administration
Pamidronate (Aredia®) Novartis	For the treatment of breast cancer that has spread to the bones.	Abdominal cramps, nausea, gastrointestinal bleeding, irregular heart beat.	Injection (IV)
Raloxifene (Evista®) Eli Lilly	Prevention of osteoporosis in postmenopausal women. Currently being tested in clinical trials for prevention and treatment of breast cancer.	Pulmonary embolism, hot flashes, chest pain, leg cramps, migraines, nausea, vomiting.	Oral (tablet)
Tamoxifen (Novadex®) AstraZeneca Pharmaceuticals	For the prevention and treatment of advanced, estrogen positive breast cancer in postmenopausal women.	Nausea, vomiting, weight gain, hot flashes, increased bone and tumor pain, blood clots, uterine cancer, cataracts, vaginal dryness or discharge.	Oral (tablet)
Thiotepa (Thioplex®) Immunex	For the palliative treatment of breast cancer.	Nausea, vomiting, anemia, hair loss.	Injection (IV)
Toremifene (Fareston®) Orion Corporation	For the treatment of metastatic breast cancer in post-menopausal estrogen-receptor positive women.	Blurred vision, menstrual changes, fatigue, heart failure, blood clots.	Oral (tablet)

Drug (Trade Name) Manufacturer	Indications	Possible Side Effects	Method of Administration
Trastuzumab (Herceptin®) Genentech	For the treatment of metastatic breast cancer which exhibits excessive amounts of the HER2 oncogene.	Heart failure, back pain, fever, chills, headache, rash, weakness, nausea, vomiting, diarrhea, hypersensitivity.	Injection (IV)
Vinblastine (Velban®) Eli Lilly	For the treatment of metastatic breast cancer.	Hair loss, heart failure, strokes, shortness of breath, inflammation of the vein.	Injection (IV)
Vinorelbine (Navelbine®) Glaxo SmithKline	For the treatment of metastatic breast cancer.	Chest pain, deep tendon reflexes, tumor pain, jaw pain, peripheral neuropathy, inflammation of the vein, fatigue, back pain.	Injection (IV)

* The side effects listed in Appendix I are not all-inclusive. Nearly all cancer drugs cause suppression of blood counts (anemia), resulting in an increased susceptibility to develop infections and fatigue. It is important to report any symptoms to your healthcare team.

Appendix II

Common Anti-Nausea Medications

Drug (Trade Name) Manufacturer	Indications	Possible Side Effects	Method of Administration
Dolasetron (Anzemet®) Aventis Pharmaceuticals	Prevent/treat nausea and vomiting following chemotherapy/surgery.	Irregular heartbeat, diarrhea, abdominal pain, headache.	Oral (tablet) Injection (IV)
Granisetron (Kytril®) Glaxo SmithKline	Prevent/treat nausea and vomiting following chemotherapy/surgery.	Headaches, constipation, anemia.	Oral (tablet) Injection (IV)
Ondansetron (Zofran®) Glaxo SmithKline	Prevent/treat nausea and vomiting following chemotherapy/surgery.	Headaches, fatigue, diarrhea, constipation, muscle pain.	Oral (tablet) Injection (IV)
Dexamethasone (generic)	To prevent delayed-onset nausea and vomiting from chemotherapy.	Irregular heartbeat, euphoria, insominia, abdominal pain, hyperglycemia, irritability, edema.	Oral (suspension and tablet), Injection (IV)
Metoclopramide (generic)	To treat breakthrough and delayed nausea and vomiting that may occur from chemotherapy.	Restlessness, seizures, abdominal pain, diarrhea, sedation.	Oral (suspension and tablet), Injection (IV)

Appendix III

Clinical Guidelines for Practitioners

BREAST DISEASE:
CLINICAL GUIDELINES
FOR PRACTITIONERS

2001

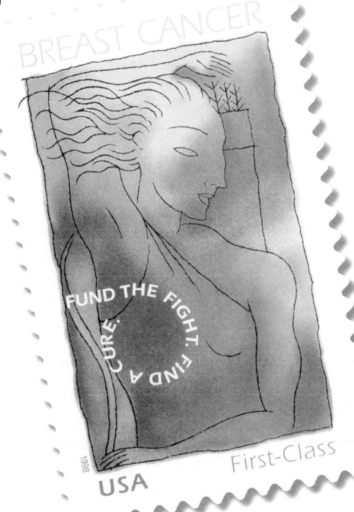

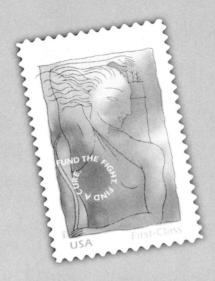

The Breast Cancer Research Stamp (BCRS) is the first-ever semipostal issued by the United States Postal Service (USPS). It is the result of the authors extensive lobbying of the United States Congress to issue a public law, authorizing the USPS to print the stamp. To date over 350 million stamps have been sold, raising $25 million for research.

Designed by Whitney Sherman, the stamp depicts Diana Artemus the Roman mythological protector of women. Diana is reaching for a bow in her quiver to fend off an enemy—in this case, breast cancer. The position she assumes is that for breast self-examination and mammography—both important tools for early detection. The rainbow of colors represents the fact that the disease is one which affects women of all colors. In addition, the rainbow is the traditional symbol for hope—a hope for the cure.

The stamps are available for purchase at all U.S. post offices and online at www.stampsonline.com. Further information is available at www.curebreastcancer.org.

TABLE OF CONTENTS

The purpose of the clinical guidelines for the management of diseases of the breast is threefold:

1) Decrease patient anxiety generated by an unnecessary referral
2) Decrease improper utilization of facilities, tests and consultants, and
3) Increase accessibility for patients requiring comprehensive evaluation/intervention

This manual is intended to provide practitioners with the information necessary to properly determine **when to refer** a patient with a breast complaint to the Breast Health Center or a surgeon.

The topics discussed, with appropriate diagnostic algorithms, are:

1) Mastalgia (Breast Pain)
2) Nipple Discharge
3) Breast Mass–Non-Dominant (Thickening, Asymmetric Nodularity)
4) Breast Mass–Dominant, Premenopausal
5) Breast Mass–Dominant, Postmenopausal
6) Skin Changes/Nipple Retraction
7) Gynecomastia
8) Breast Implant Concerns–Cosmetic
9) Breast Implant Concerns–Reconstructive
10) Macromastia/Breast Hyperplasia
11) Breast Cancer Surveillance Guidelines

These are **only** guidelines; each patient may have extenuating circumstances or present with a particular dilemma. **Anyone** should be referred if the level of concern exceeds the pathways presented, or the appropriate level of evaluation for consultation has been reached.

Questions/suggestions/comments? Contact us at:

The Breast Health Center
Kaiser Permanente
1650 Response Road, Suite 3A
Sacramento, CA 95815

(916) 614-KARE (5273), *Fax:* (916) 614-5124

THE WOMAN AT HIGH RISK:
AN IMPORTANT DEFINITION

- Previous History of Breast or Ovarian Cancer

- Family History of Breast Cancer

  Mother ⎤
  Sister   ⎬— Particularly if diagnosed at age < 50
  Daughter ⎦

- Previous Biopsy with a Pathologic Diagnosis of:

  Atypical ductal hyperplasia
  Lobular carcinoma-in-situ

- Previous History of Chest or Cervical Radiation Therapy

SCREENING GUIDELINES FOR BREAST CANCER DETECTION

HIGH RISK

Age	Mammography	Clinical Breast Exam
20–34	Not Recommended	With Routine Gyn Exam
40–74	Yearly	Yearly
>75	Physician Recommended/ Patient Desire	Yearly

AVERAGE RISK*

Age	Mammography	Clinical Breast Exam
20–39	Not Recommended* (Baseline at 35)	With Routine Gyn Exam
40–74	Yearly	Yearly
>75	Physician Recommended/ Patient Desire	Yearly

Refers to women who do not have the risk factors described above. Most females are average risk.

Note: Mammographic screening starts at age 35 or 5 years prior to the youngest 1st degree relative diagnosed with breast or ovarian cancer (i.e. if a 1st degree relative was diagnosed at age 32, screening is indicated at age 27). BSE recommended monthly in all patients. Instruction in BSE is available at most Breast Health Centers.

MASTALGIA (BREAST PAIN)

Mastalgia is the most common breast-related complaint at primary care clinics as well as breast referral centers. Two-thirds of patients complain of breast pain; more than 50% are cyclic in nature.

	CYCLIC (MENSTRUAL RELATED)	NONCYCLIC
Location	Bilateral	Unilateral
Character	Diffuse, Dull, Full, Aching, Heavy	Localized, Sharp, Throbbing, Stabbing, Burning

Fibrocystic changes represent the most common cause of cyclic breast pain. Non-cyclic causes include cervical radiculitis, intercostal neuritis, shingles, Tietze's Syndrome (costochondritis), mastitis/abscess, Mondor's disease, trauma, post radiation syndrome and **rarely** cancer. Each of these origins of pain can be well characterized, and may pinpoint the etiology.

ETIOLOGY	CHARACTERISTICS
Fibrocystic Disease	Cyclic (increases as menses approach), dull, full, aching, heavy
Cervical Radiculitis	Intermittent, sharp, stabbing, radiating
Intercostal Neuritis	Intermittent, sharp, stabbing, radiating, often arising at a site of previous scarring, or a specific pressure point (e.g. at site of the wire in underwire bras.)
Shingles	Like radiculitis, plus the characteristic rash
Tietze's Syndrome (costochondritis)	Point tenderness at the costochondral junction (reproducible with pressure at the site)
Mastitis/Abscess	Erythema, aching, throbbing, systemic signs of infection
Mondor's Disease	Superficial thrombophlebitis of the breast presenting as a tender palpable cord
Trauma	Soreness, ecchymosis, edema (history may be remote)
Post Radiation Syndrome	Redness, constant dull ache, heaviness
Cancer	Very rarely, but if so, sharp and pinpoint

Mastalgia (Breast Pain)

History/CBE

Cyclic

Reassure: Symtomatic Tx (NSAIDs, EPO)

Repeat CBE in 3–6 months

- **Pain Resolved** → Routine F/U
- **Pain Persists** → Clinical Judgment: Reassurance/ Mammogram/ Client Preference → Mammogram (–): Danazol (If patient demands Tx)

Non-Cyclic

Mammogram/UTZ (age ≥ 35)

- **Negative** → Reassure: Symtomatic Tx (NSAIDs, EPO) → Routine F/U
- **Suspicious** → Bx: FNA/Core → (+) Surgical Referral

Protocol for Mass or Other Findings

See Appropriate Algorithm

A variety of causes have been hypothesized to explain mastalgia; all have failed to completely explain the mechanism of breast pain. Currently, the consensus of opinion favors hormonal stimulation of breast tissues resulting in nerve root irritation. Which hormones are the cause and what medications might improve the situation remain unknown.

TREATMENT

Once reassured, most women are convinced that pain is not a symptom of breast cancer. A supportive brassiere and nonsteroidal antiinflammatory drugs (NSAIDs) such as Ibuprofen usually treat the pain adequately.

If further medical therapy is desired, a four month course of evening primrose oil (EPO) may be tried. A food supplement high in essential fatty acids, EPO has been found to be effective in treating breast pain, when compared to placebo. Evening primrose oil is high in linoleic and gammalinolenic acid, two essential fatty acids. These are believed to affect prostaglandin metabolism. EPO is available over the counter for about $40 per month. The dose is six 500mg capsules per day, beginning on day 15 of the menstrual cycle, continuing until menses or every day if the breast pain is not cyclic. It has no known side effects.

Vitamin E, 400–800 iu/day has been beneficial in some women as has the addition of vitamin B_6/B_{12} complex administration daily. Discontinuation of caffeine products (i.e. coffee, tea and soft drinks) may also help decrease breast pain.

The most effective medication studied for severe mastalgia is Danazol, a testosterone derivative which may affect estrogen and testosterone levels, decreasing ovarian stimulation and lowering serum lipid levels. Side effects include weight gain and menstrual irregularities. The medication should be prescribed only as a last resort, or to those women who demand treatment, after having failed other modalities. The dose is 100–400 mg/day.

A complaint of nipple discharge is the third most feared breast symptom following pain and the finding of a 'new' lump. The **vast** majority of nipple discharges represent a benign condition and do not warrant surgical evaluation; patients can be treated with education and reassurance. Nipple discharge, regardless of character, is rarely a sympton of an underlying carcinoma. (Nipple discharge in males is more often associated with breast cancer.) Significant nipple discharge, warranting further evaluation, must fill certain criteria **prior** to referral. They must be:

1) Unilateral
2) Spontaneous
3) Persistent
4) Bloody (hemoccult positive)

TYPES OF NIPPLE DISCHARGE

Type	Characteristics
Milky	Bilateral, multiple ducts, resembles skim milk
Multicolored*	Bilateral, multiple ducts, sticky, predominantly greenish/yellow
Purulent	Unilateral, pus, pain/tenderness, signs of inflammation/infection
Clear/Watery	Unilateral, resembling a drop of water; rarely associated with cancer unless profuse and serous in nature
Bloody	Unilateral, Hemoccult/Hemostix positive. Further investigation/biopsy (areolar clean out) indicated. Most often secondary to an intraductal papilloma (benign).

May appear bloody grossly, but when spread on a tissue or gauze pad, stains brown/green, not red. Test for blood using Hemoccult or Hemostix.

Significant nipple discharge is elicited only from a single duct, not multiple ducts. A 5–10% incidence of carcinoma in patients with bloody or watery discharge has been reported.

Nipple discharges whose character suggest a fibrocystic etiology (serous, green, gray) need no further evaluation. Green, yellow or milky discharge should not be referred for ductography. Reassurance is the treatment of choice. Other etiologies are treated appropriately, i.e., elimination of medications.

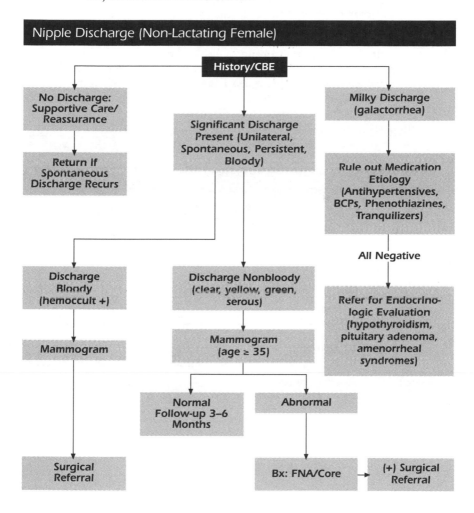

Nipple Discharge (Non-Lactating Female)

History/CBE

No Discharge: Supportive Care/ Reassurance

Return If Spontaneous Discharge Recurs

Significant Discharge Present (Unilateral, Spontaneous, Persistent, Bloody)

Milky Discharge (galactorrhea)

Rule out Medication Etiology (Antihypertensives, BCPs, Phenothiazines, Tranquilizers)

All Negative

Discharge Bloody (hemoccult +)

Mammogram

Discharge Nonbloody (clear, yellow, green, serous)

Mammogram (age ≥ 35)

Refer for Endocrinologic Evaluation (hypothyroidism, pituitary adenoma, amenorrheal syndromes)

Normal Follow-up 3–6 Months

Abnormal

Surgical Referral

Bx: FNA/Core → (+) Surgical Referral

The female with 'non-lumpy' breasts is rare. Almost all women have some element of fibrocystic disease. This condition, in reality, is not a disease at all, but represents a normal variant of breast tissue. Nonetheless, fibrocystic breasts are a major source of concern and anxiety, not only for the patient, but also for significant others as well as physicians.

Non-dominant lumps represent diffuse thickenings, areas of asymmetry and/or nodularity which are distinguishable from multiple, separate masses and/or cysts. The vast majority of such findings are benign: reassurance, education and instruction in the proper technique of Breast Self Exam is the only required treatment. The most significant risk factor for the development of breast cancer is age, therefore the evaluation of non-dominant masses in pre and post-menopausal patients varies.

The Non Dominant Mass (Asymmetric Thickening)

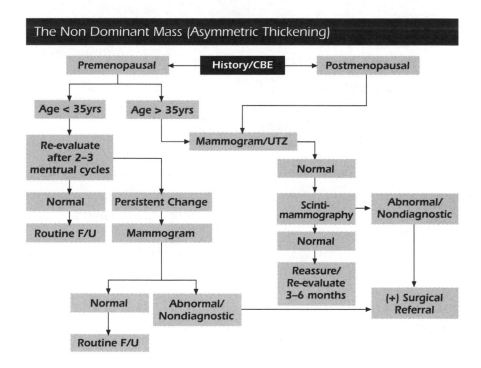

Note: An appropriate indication for biopsy is the patient's request, if for nothing else, reassurance.

THE DOMINANT MASS

Perhaps no other finding raises more fear in a female than the discovery of a 'lump' in the breast. A dominant mass is distinct and persists through multiple menstrual cycles. While the majority of these 'lumps' are benign, solitary masses warrant further evaluation. Non-suspicious lumps usually represent a cyst or fibroadenoma and are characterized by pain, easy mobility and cyclic variation in size and tenderness. Suspicious lumps are generally non-tender, do not change with menses, continue to grow and may be fixed (nonmobile). Since the most significant risk factor for the development of breast cancer is age, the evaluation of dominant masses in pre and post-menopausal patients varies.

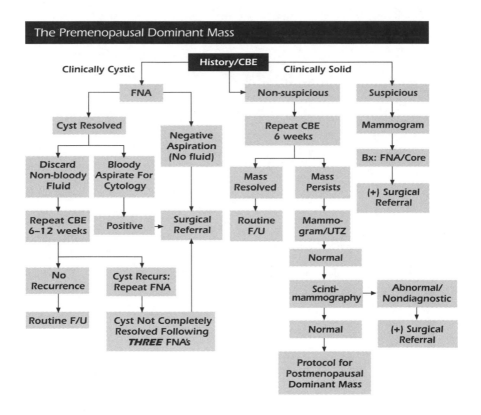

The Premenopausal Dominant Mass

The Postmenopausal Dominant Mass

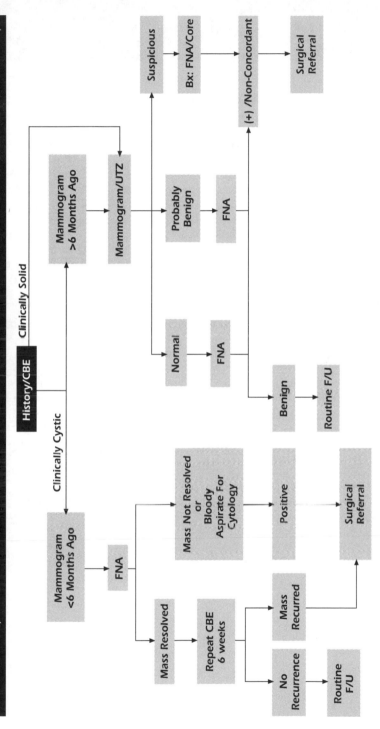

Skin Changes (redness, retraction, orange-peel (peau d'orange) appearance with or without accompanying nipple retraction, if unilateral and unexplained (localized infection, insect bites, trauma, etc.) represents an ominous finding. The onset of symptoms is particularly important: a long standing history of nipple retraction is insignificant, particularly if it is bilateral. Further, if manipulation of the nipple results in eversion, a benign etiology is favored.

Inflammation, unresponsive to antibiotics and local therapy, requires surgical referral. Mammography, even if interpreted as normal, does not preclude further investigation in the patient with ongoing skin changes which are refractile to conservative measures.

Inflammatory carcinoma has a poor prognosis. Suspicion for this condition should be very high in the presence of:

1) breast edema (skin dimpling or peau d'orange)
2) nipple retraction/deviation
3) unilateral redness without response to conservative treatment and an obvious etiology

Paget's disease is a unique presentation of breast cancer and is characterized by crusting or scaling of the nipple, unresponsive to a short course of steroids, antibiotics or local therapy. **Areolar** scaling or eczema **without** nipple involvement is not a sign of Paget's disease. Erythema associated with Paget's disease is an inflammatory response to cancer cells which are present. Topical steroids may cause apparent resolution of the skin condition, but they quickly re-occur when the steroids are discontinued. In these cases, a biopsy of the involved skin is indicated.

The significance of Paget's disease of the breast lies in the fact that it is always associated with an underlying carcinoma of the breast. Such carcinomas may be premalignant (in-situ) or malignant (invasive). A normal mammogram, in such a setting, does not preclude the presence of an underlying cancerous condition.

Breast Skin Changes/Nipple Retraction

History/CBE → **Suspicious Skin Changes/Nipple Retraction**

Recent Onset (<6months)

- **Yes**
  - **Bilateral?**
    - **No**
      - **Mass**
        - **No** → **Mammogram** → **Benign** → **Repeat CBE 3 Months**
          - **Suspicious**
          - **Unresolved**
          - **F/U or Bx, Based on Clinical Judgement/Client Preference**
          - **Resolved** → **Routine F/U**
        - **Yes** → **See protocol for evaluation of mass**
      - **Crusty Nipple Changes, Consistent with Pagets Disease**
        - **Mammogram**
        - **Surgical Referral**
    - **Yes**
      - **Inflammatory Skin Changes**
        - **10 Days of Antibiotics**
        - **Repeat CBE**
          - **Symptoms Not Resolved** → **Mammogram** → **Surgical Referral**
          - **Symptoms Resolved** → **Routine F/U**

- **No** → **Repeat CBE Within 3 Months**
  - **Not Resolved** → (Mammogram / Surgical Referral)
  - **Resolved** → **Routine F/U**

Routine F/U

Gynecomastia represents an increase in breast ductal and connective tissue in males. It is most often benign and peaks in two age groups: the adolescent and those over fifty. The evaluation of gynecomastia is directed by the age group in which the condition presents. It is most often unilateral and painful.

Pseudogynecomastia is a condition that clinically mimics gynecomastica. Instead of excess breast tissue, excess fat is present. This fat is amenable to removal by liposuction whereas 'true' gynecomastia is not. Referral to Plastic Surgery is based on: breast size sufficient to simulate a 'B' cup bra or gross asymmetry.

Breast cancer in males is rare (approximately 1,500 cases per year in the *United States*).

CAUSES OF GYNECOMASTIA

Idiopathic	• Etiology unknown
Drug Induced	• Estrogens/Androgens • Alcohol • Cimetidine • Marijuana • Digoxin • Tricyclic/Anti- • Antihypertensives depressants • Isoniazid • Heroin
Hepatic Failure	
Testosterone Deficiency	• Klinefelter's Syndrome • Testicular Feminization
Thyrotoxicosis	• Hyperfunctioning Thyroid
Malignancy	• Testicular • Adrenal • Bronchogenic • Pituitary

Gynecomastia

History/CBE

Adolescent

Testicular Exam
- Normal → Reassure Repeat CBE 6 months → Persistent/Increased Breast Tissue → R/O Drug Abuse Repeat CBE 6 Months → Persistent (With Emotional/Physical Embarrassment) → Plastic Surgery Referral
- Atrophy/Asymmetry Abnormal → Endocrine Evaluation

Reassure Repeat CBE 6 months

>50 years age

Testicular Exam, CXR, LFT's Review Medications → No Obvious Etiology → Mammogram

Mammogram →
- Suspicious, Non-Concordant → Bx: FNA/Core → (+), Non-Concordant → Surgical Referral
- Consistent with Gynecomastia → Reassure Repeat CBE 6 months → Persistent, Painful → Surgical Referral

Currently, over two million women in the United States have breast implants. They have been inserted for one of three reasons: to cosmetically augment breasts, to reconstruct breasts after mastectomy, or to augment one breast as a method to restore symmetry. Currently most health plans will cover the **removal** of implants placed for cosmetic reasons. Removal and replacement for reconstructive or asymmetric cases are also covered benefits. However most health plans do **not replace** implants for **cosmetic** reasons. Patients with cosmetic breast augmentation requesting **replacement** should be referred to their original Plastic Surgeon.

Breast implants are filled with either saline or silicone. Except for rupture and/or leakage, both may cause similar problems. The most common complaints associated with breast implants are capsular contracture with or without pain, adjacent masses or lumps, rupture or leakage, abnormal findings on mammography and anxiety regarding immune dysfunction. Most of these problems will require consultation with a Plastic Surgeon for evaluation and treatment. Recent studies have failed to demonstrate an increased risk for the development of connective tissue disorders in patients with implants. Only reassurance is required. Similarly, the incidence of breast cancer does not increase with the presence of breast implants. Rate of implant rupture appears to correlate with the age of the implant.

Mammograms of the implanted breast require special techniques for optimal visualization. The presence of breast implants should be noted on the radiology request form. A CT scan is the current recommendation to rule out implant leakage or rupture. An MRI will occassionally be needed to confirm the diagnosis.

Cosmetic Breast Implant Concerns

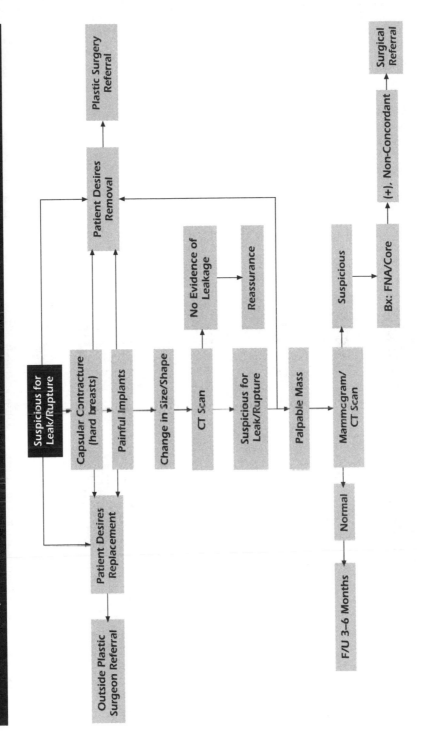

Reconstructive Breast Implant Concerns

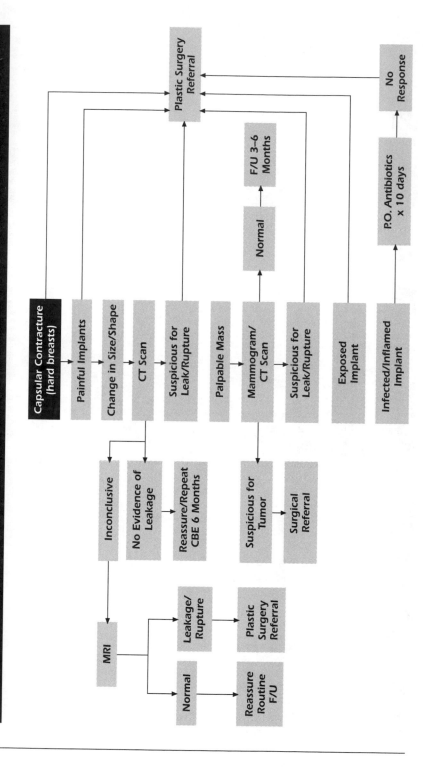

Patients presenting with uncomfortably large breasts can often be helped by breast reduction surgery, regardless of age. It should be emphasized that large breasts are reduced to smaller breasts at the expense of leaving scars, occasionally accompanied by chronic pain. In addition, the patient should be warned that breast reduction surgery may alter the baseline values of BSE, CBE and routine mammography for surveillance.

Certain criteria should be met prior to referral for reduction mammoplasty. The patients' breasts should be a 'D' cup or larger. They should have symptoms such as back, neck or shoulder pain, shoulder grooving from bra straps, significant submammary intertrigo, and interference with physical activities such as running. Candidates should be within twenty percent of their ideal weight **prior** to consultation.

Most patients are satisfied after surgery but there are risks and limitations that the Plastic Surgeon will discuss with the patient at consultation.

DESIRABLE WEIGHTS FOR WOMEN ACCORDING TO HEIGHT, AGE 25 AND OVER

Height		Weight	20% Over
Feet	Inches	Pounds	Pounds
4	10	<119	~143
4	11	<122	~147
5	0	<125	~150
5	1	<128	~154
5	2	<131	~157
5	3	<134	~161
5	4	<138	~166
5	5	<142	~171
5	6	<146	~175
5	7	<150	~180
5	8	<154	~185
5	9	<158	~190
5	10	<163	~195
5	11	<168	~202
6	0	<173	~208

Macromastia/Breast Hyperplasia

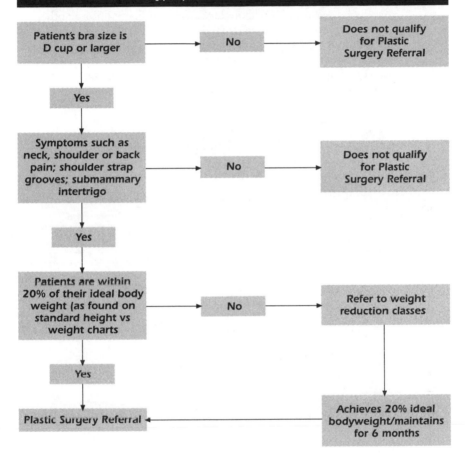

Patient's bra size is D cup or larger → **No** → Does not qualify for Plastic Surgery Referral

↓ Yes

Symptoms such as neck, shoulder or back pain; shoulder strap grooves; submammary intertrigo → **No** → Does not qualify for Plastic Surgery Referral

↓ Yes

Patients are within 20% of their ideal body weight (as found on standard height vs weight charts → **No** → Refer to weight reduction classes

↓ Yes

Plastic Surgery Referral ← Achieves 20% ideal bodyweight/maintains for 6 months

Once diagnosed with breast cancer, the patient is forever concerned about the possibility of recurrence. Despite maximal therapy, every new ache and pain is attributed to a recurrence, until proven otherwise. No **new** symptom (i.e., new lump in axilla, mass or rash at incision site) should be ignored, and clinical judgment is crucial in the evaluation of any such complaints.

As a general guideline for routine surveillance (in addition to monthly BSE), the following recommendations are made:

BREAST CANCER SURVEILLANCE GUIDELINES

Years 1 & 2	CBE	Mammogram (Affected Breast)	Mammogram Bilateral
3 Months	■		
6	■	■	
12	■		■
18	■	■	
24	■		■

Years 3–5	CBE	Mammogram Bilateral
6 Months	■	
12	■	■

> 5 Years	CBE	Mammogram Bilateral
	Annual	Annual

Patients with lumpectomies should do bilateral breast exams **monthly.** Mastectomy patients should examine the incision site visually and by palpation for any nodules, skin changes or retraction in the area, and should perform BSE on the contralateral side.

The American Society of Clinical Oncology currently finds that data are insufficient to recommend routine CXR, CBCs, bone scans, liver ultrasounds or CT scans in the absence of specific complaints or symptoms. Tumor marker evaluation is currently not indicated.

EVALUATION OF SUSPECTED RECURRENCE

Hematologic:

- CBC
- LFT's

Radiologic:

- Chest X-Ray
- X-Rays of symptomatic bones or those positive on nuclear scan
- CT Scan
- MRI of symptomatic area

Surgical:

- Bx suspected area

GLOSSARY OF ABBREVIATIONS

BSE .... Breast Self Exam

Bx .... Biopsy

CBC .... Complete Blood Count

CBE .... Clinical Breast Exam

Concordant .... Agrees with previous study

CT Scan .... Computerized Oxical Tomography

EPO .... Evening Primrose Oil

FNA...................................... Fine needle aspiration

F/U .... Follow-up

LFT's .... Liver Function Tests

MRI...................................... Magnetic Resonance Imaging

Non-Concordant .... Disagrees with previous study
.... or clinical impressions

R/O .... Rule Out

Tx .... Treatment

UTZ .... Ultrasound

Appendix IV

Glossary of Breast Cancer Terms

Appendix IV

Glossary of Breast Cancer Terms

A

Adenoma: A noncancerous tumor.

Adjuvant therapy: Treatment given in addition to the primary treatment to enhance the effectiveness of the primary treatment.

Anemia: A decrease in the normal amount of red blood cells.

Angiogenesis: Blood vessel formation, which usually accompanies the growth of malignant tissue.

Antibiotics: Drugs used to treat infection.

Antibody: A protein produced by certain white blood cells in response to a foreign substance (antigen). Each antibody can bind only to a specific antigen. The purpose of this binding is to help destroy the antigen. Antibodies can work in several ways; some antibodies disable antigens directly, others make the antigen more vulnerable to destruction by white blood cells.

Antigen: Any foreign or "non-self" substance that, when introduced into the body, causes the immune system to create an antibody.

Areola: The area of dark-colored skin that surrounds the nipple.

Aspiration: Removal of fluid from a lump, often a cyst, with a needle and a syringe.

Asymptomatic: Presenting no signs or symptoms of disease.

Atypical hyperplasia: A benign (noncancerous) condition in which there are larger numbers of cells than normal.

Axilla: The underarm.

Axillary: Pertaining to the underarm.

Axillary dissection: Surgery to remove lymph nodes under the arm.

B

Benign: Not cancerous; does not invade nearby tissue or spread to other parts of the body.

Beta-carotene: A substance from which vitamin A is formed; a precursor of vitamin A.

Bilateral: Affecting both sides of the body.

Biological response modifiers: Substances that stimulate the body's response to infection and disease. The body naturally produces small amounts of these substances. Scientists can produce some of them in the laboratory in large amounts and use them in cancer treatment.

Biological therapy: The use of the body's immune system, either directly or indirectly, to fight cancer or to lessen side effects that may be caused by some cancer treatments. Also known as immunotherapy, biotherapy, or biological response modifier therapy.

Biopsy: The removal of a piece of tissue, which is then examined under a microscope to check for cancer cells.

Bone marrow: The soft, spongy tissue in the center of large bones that produces white blood cells, red blood cells, and platelets.

Bone scan: A technique to create images of bones on a computer screen or on film. A small amount of radioactive material is injected into a vein. It collects in the bones, especially in abnormal areas, and is detected by a scanner.

BRCA1: A gene located on chromosome 17 that normally helps to restrain cell growth. Inheriting an altered version of BRCA1 predisposes an individual to breast, ovarian, and prostate cancer.

BRCA2: A gene located on chromosome 13 that normally helps to restrain cell growth. Inheriting an altered version of BRCA2 predisposes an individual to breast, ovarian, and prostate cancer.

Breast reconstruction: Surgery to rebuild a breast following a mastectomy.

C

Calcium: A mineral found mainly in the hard part of bones.

Cancer/carcinoma: A term for diseases in which abnormal cells divide without control. Cancer cells can invade nearby tissues and can spread through the bloodstream and lymphatic system to other parts of the body.

Carcinogen: Any substance that is known to cause cancer.

Carcinoma in situ: Cancer that involves only the cells in which it began and does not have the potential to spread to other tissues.

Cell: The basic unit of any living organism.

Chemoprevention: The use of natural or laboratory-made substances to try to prevent cancer.

Chemotherapy: Treatment with anticancer drugs.

Chromosome: Part of a cell that contains genetic information. Normally, human cells contain 46 chromosomes that appear as a long thread inside the cell.

Clinical trials: Research studies that involve patients. Each study is carefully designed to find better ways to prevent, detect, diagnose or treat cancer.

Combination chemotherapy: Treatment in which two or more chemicals are used to obtain more effective results.

Computed tomography: An x-ray procedure that uses a computer to produce a detailed picture of a cross section of the body; also called a CAT or CT scan. Used mostly for staging, not diagnosis.

Cyst: A sac or capsule filled with fluid.

D

Differentiation: In cancer, refers to how mature (developed) the cancer cells are in a tumor. Differentiated tumor cells resemble normal cells and grow at a slower rate than undifferentiated tumor cells, which lack the structure and function of normal cells and grow at a more rapid rate.

DNA (deoxyribonucleic acid): The substance of heredity; a large molecule that carries the genetic information that cells need to replicate and produce proteins.

Duct: A tube through which body fluids pass.

Ductal carcinoma in situ: Abnormal cells that involve only the lining of a duct. The cells have not spread outside the duct to other parts of the body, nor do they have the potential to spread to distant organs.

E

Encapsulated: The tumor remains in a compact form, confined to a specific area.

Enzyme: A substance that affects the rate at which chemical changes take place in the body.

Estrogen: The main female hormone, produced primarily by the ovaries.

External radiation: Radiation therapy that uses a machine to aim high-energy x-rays at a cancerous growth in the body.

F

Fertility: The ability to get pregnant.

Fluorouracil: An anticancer drug. Its chemical name is 5-fluorouracil, commonly called 5-FU.

Fractionation: Dividing the total dose of radiation therapy into several smaller, equal doses delivered over a period of time.

G

Gene: The basic unit of heredity found in all cells of the body.

Gene therapy: Treatment that alters genes (the basic units of heredity found in all cells of the body). In studies of gene therapy for cancer, researchers are trying to improve the body's natural ability to fight the disease or to make the tumor more sensitive to other kinds of therapy.

Genetic: Inherited; having to do with information that is passed from parents to children through DNA in the genes.

Gland: An organ that produces and releases one or more substances for use in the body. Some glands produce fluids that affect tissues or organs. Others produce hormones or participate in blood production.

Grade: Describes how closely a cancer resembles normal tissue of the same type, and the cancer's probable rate of growth.

Grading: A system for classifying cancer cells in terms of how malignant or aggressive they appear microscopically. The grading of a tumor indicates how quickly cancer cells are likely to spread and plays an important role in treatment decisions.

H

Hair follicles: The sacs in the scalp from which hair grows.

Hematogenous: Orginating in the blood, or disseminated by the circulation or through the bloodstream.

HER-2/neu: An oncogene found in some breast and ovarian cancer patients that is associated with a poor prognosis due to increased risk of recurrence.

Hormonal therapy: Treatment that prevents certain cancers from getting the hormones they need to grow.

Hormone receptor test: A test to measure the amount of certain proteins, called hormone receptors, in breast cancer tissue. Hormones can attach to these proteins. A high level of hormone receptors means that the hormones probably help the cancer grow.

Hormones: Chemicals produced by glands in the body that control the actions of certain cells or organs.

I

Immune system: The complex group of organs and cells that defends the body against infection or disease.

Immunosuppression: The use of drugs to suppress or interfere with the body's immune system and therefore impact its ability to fight infections or disease.

Immunotherapy: Treatment that uses the body's natural defenses to fight cancer. Also called biological therapy.

Inflammatory breast cancer: A rare type of breast cancer in which cancer cells block the lymph vessels in the skin of the breast. The breast becomes red, swollen, and warm, and the skin of the breast may appear pitted or have ridges. Inflammatory breast cancer represents advanced-stage disease.

Intravenous: Injected in a vein. Also called an IV.

Invasion: As related to cancer, the spread of cancer cells into healthy tissues adjacent to the tumor.

Invasive (infiltrating) cancer/carcinoma: Cancer that has spread beyond the layer of tissue in which it developed.

L

Lobular carcinoma in situ: Abnormal cells in the lobules of the breast. This condition does not become invasive cancer. However, having lobular carcinoma-in-situ is a sign that a woman has an increased risk of developing breast cancer. Also called LCIS.

Lumpectomy: Surgery to remove only the cancerous breast lump; usually followed by radiation therapy.

Lymph: The colorless fluid that travels through the lymphatic system and carries cells that help fight infection and disease.

Lymph nodes: Small organs located along the channels of the lymphatic system. The lymph nodes store special cells that can trap bacteria or cancer cells traveling through the body in the lymph. Clusters of lymph nodes are found in the underarms, groin, neck, chest, and abdomen. Also called lymph glands.

Lymphedema: A condition in which excess fluid collects in the soft tissues and causes swelling. It may occur in the arm or leg after lymph vessels or lymph nodes in the underarm or groin are removed, or become blocked by cancer cells.

M

Macrocalcifications: Tiny deposits of calcium in the breast detected on a mammogram. A cluster of these small specks of calcium likely represent benign (non-cancerous) changes in the breast due to the normal aging process.

Magnetic resonance imaging: A procedure in which a magnet, linked to a computer, is used to create detailed pictures of areas inside the body. Also called an MRI.

Malignant: Cancerous; can invade nearby tissue and spread to other parts of the body.

Mammogram: An x-ray of the breast.

Mammography: The use of x-rays to create a picture of the breast.

Mammotome®: A minimally invasive alternative to open surgical biopsy which uses a unique vacuum-assisted technique to provide tissue samples of breast abnormalities.

Mastectomy: Surgery to remove the breast (or as much of the breast as possible).

Menopause: The time in a woman's life when menstrual periods cease and female hormone levels drop dramatically.

Menstrual cycle: The hormone changes that lead up to a woman's having a period. For most women, one cycle takes 28 days.

Metastasize: To spread from one part of the body to another. When cancer cells metastasize and form secondary tumors, the cells in the metastatic tumor are like those in the original (primary) tumor.

Microcalcifications: Tiny deposits of calcium in the breast detected on a mammogram. A cluster of these small specks of calcium may indicate that an early cancer is present.

Monoclonal antibodies: Substances that can locate and bind to cancer cells wherever they are in the body. They can be used alone, or they can be used to deliver drugs, toxins, or radioactive material directly to tumor cells.

O

Oncogene: The part of the cell that normally directs cell growth, but which can also promote or allow the uncontrolled growth of cancer if damaged (mutated) by exposure to carcinogens, or acquired as an inherited defect.

Oncologist: A doctor who specializes in the medical treatment of cancer. Some oncologists specialize in a particular type of cancer treatment (e.g., a radiation oncologist treats cancers with radiation).

Ovaries: The pair of female reproductive glands in which the ova (eggs) are formed.

P

Palliation: Treatment that does not alter the course of a disease, but only eases symptoms and improves the quality of life.

Pathologist: A doctor who identifies a disease by studying the cells and tissues under a microscope.

Positron emission tomography scan: For this type of scan, a person is given a substance that reacts with tissues in the body to release protons (parts of an atom). Through measuring the different amounts of protons released by healthy and cancerous tissues, a computer creates a picture of the inside of the body. Also called a PET scan.

Precancerous: A term used to describe a condition that may or is likely to become a "real" cancer, with the potential to invade nearby organs or travel to distant organs (metastasize).

Progesterone: The second dominant female hormone (after estrogen).

Prognosis: The probable outcome or course of a disease.

R

R2 ImageChecker: A computerized system capable of digitizing mammographic images, identifying possible abnormalities missed by a radiologist.

Radiation therapy: Treatment with high-energy x-rays to kill cancer cells. Also called radiotherapy.

Recurrence: The reappearance of cancer cells at the same (primary) site or in a distant location.

Remission: Disappearance of the signs and symptoms of cancer. When this happens, the disease is said to be "in remission."

Resection: Surgical removal of part of an organ.

Risk factor: Something that increases the chance of developing a disease.

S

Salpingo-oophorectomy: Surgical removal of the fallopian tubes and ovaries.

Scintimammography: A breast imaging technique that tracks radio-active tracers as they concentrate in cancer cells.

Screening: Checking for a disease when there are no symptoms.

Side effects: Problems that occur when treatment affects healthy cells. Common side effects of cancer treatment are fatigue, nausea, vomiting, decreased blood cell counts, hair loss, and an increased incidence of infections.

Staging: The method used to determine the extent of a cancer, especially whether it has spread from its original site to other parts of the body.

Stereotaxis: Use of a computer and imaging devices to create three-dimensional pictures. This method can be used to direct a biopsy or the application of external radiation.

Steroids: Drugs used to relieve swelling and inflammation.

Systemic therapy: Treatment that uses substances that travel through the bloodstream, reaching and affecting cancer cells all over the body.

T

Testosterone: The dominant male sex hormone.

Tumor marker: A substance in blood or other body fluids that may suggest that a person has cancer.

U

Ultrasound: A test that bounces sound waves off tissues and internal organs and changes the echoes into pictures (sonograms). Tissues of different densities reflect sound waves differently.

My Notes

"Terms I Need To Understand Better"
(And to ask my doctor or nurse about!)

_____

_____

_____

_____

_____

_____

_____

_____

_____

_____

_____

_____

_____

Appendix V

Off the Bookshelf

Appendix V

Off the Bookshelf

Affirmations, Meditations and Encouragements for Women Living with Breast Cancer, Linda Dackman

After Cancer, A Guide to Your New Life, Wendy S.Harpham. M.D.

A Woman's Decision: Breast Care, Treatment and Reconstruction, Karen Berger and John Bostwick III, M.D.

Be A Survivor: Your Guide to Breast Cancer Treatment, Vladimir Lange, M.D.

Beautiful Again: Restoring Your Image and Enhancing Body Changes, Jan Willis

Be Prepared: The Complete Financial, Legal and Practical Guide for Living with a Life-Challenging Condition, David S. Landay

Beauty and Cancer, Looking and Feeling Your Best, Diane Doan Noyes and Peggy Mellody, R.N.

Bosom Buddies, Rosie O'Donnell and Deborah Axelrod, M.D., F.A.C.S.

Breast Cancer: A Family Survival Guide, Lucille M. Penderson and Janet M. Trig

Breast Cancer? Let Me Check My Schedule!, D. Cederberg, D. Davidson, et. al.

Breast Cancer: Reducing Your Risk (If It Runs In Your Family), M.D. Eades

Breast Cancer Survivor's Club, A Nurse's Experience, Lillie Shockney, R.N.

Breast Cancer: The Complete Guide, Yashar Hirshaut, M.D. and Peter Pressman, M.D.

Cancer Clinical Trials: Experimental Treatments and How They Can Help You, Robert Finn

Celebrating Life, Sylvia Dunnavant

Chemotherapy Gives New Meaning to a Bad Hair Day, Eileen Marin

Coping with Chemotherapy, Nancy Bruning

Coping When A Parent Has Cancer, Linda Strauss

Dancing in Limbo, Making Sense of Life After Cancer, Glenna Halvorson-Boyd and Lisa K. Hunter

Diagnosis Cancer, Your Guide Through the First Few Months, Wendy Schlessel Harpham, M.D.

Dr. Susan Love's Breast Book, Susan Love, M.D.

Everyone's Guide to Cancer Therapy, Malin Dollinger, M.D., Ernest H. Rosenbaum, M.D., and Greg Cable

Examining Myself, Musa Mayer

Fine Black Lines: Reflections on Facing Cancer, Fear and Loneliness, Lois Tschetter Hjelmstad

Guide for Cancer Supporters, Annette and Richard Bloch

Healing, A Woman's Guide to Recovery After Mastectomy, by Rosalind Delores Benedet, N.P., M.S.N.

Helping Your Mate Face Breast Cancer: Tips for Becoming an Effective Support Partner, Judy C. Kneece, R.N., OCN

Hope is Contagious – The Breast Cancer Treatment Survival Handbook, Margit Esser Porter

Intimacy: Living as a Woman After Cancer, Jacquelyn Johnson

In Touch With Your Breasts, James Davidson, M.D. and Jan Winebrenner

Invisible Scars: A Guide to Coping with the Emotional Impact of Breast Cancer, Mimi Greenberg, Ph.D.

Journey Unknown, Margaret Phalor Barnhart

Living Beyond Breast Cancer, Marisa C. Weiss and Ellen Weiss

Living in the Postmastectomy Body: Learning to Live and Love Your Body Again, Becky Zuchweiler, M.S., R.N

Love, Judy: Letters of Hope and Healing for Women with Breast Cancer, Judy Hart

Lymphedema, A Breast Cancer Patient's Guide to Prevention and Healing, Jeannie Burt and Gwen White

Man to Man: When the Woman You Love Has Breast Cancer, Andy Murcia and Bob Stewart

Moms Don't Get Sick, Pat Brack

My Mother's Breast: Daughters Face Their Mother's Cancer, Laurie Tarkan

Nutrition for the Chemotherapy Patient, Janet Ramstack, Ph.D. and Ernest H. Rosenbaum, M.D.

Once Upon A Hopeful Night, Risa Yaffe

Our Family Has Cancer, Too!, Christine Clifford

Paper Chain, C. Blake, E. Blanchard and K. Parkinson

Relaxation and Stress Reduction Workbook, Martha Davis, Elizabeth Robbins Eshelman, and Matthew McKay

Spinning Straw Into Gold, Ronnie Kaye

Straight from the Heart: Letters of Hope and Inspiration from Survivors of Breast Cancer, Ina Yalof

Straight Talk about Breast Cancer, Suzanne W. Braddock, M.D., Jane Kercher, M.D., et. al.

The Activist Cancer Patient, Beverly Zakarian

The Breast Cancer Companion, Kathy LaTour

The Breast Cancer Handbook, Joan Swirsky and Barbara Balaban

The Breast Cancer Survival Manual, John Link, M.D.

The Cancer Conquerer, Greg Anderson

The Not-So-Scary Breast Cancer Book, Carolyn Ingram, Ed.D and Leslie Ingram Gebhart, M.A

The Race is Run One Step at a Time, Nancy Brinker

The Wellness Community Guide to Fighting for Recovery from Cancer, Harold H. Benjamin, Ph.D.

To Be Alive, A Woman's Guide to a Full Life After Cancer, Carolyn D. Runowicz, M.D. and Donna Haupt

Upfront – Sex and the Post-Mastectomy Woman, Linda Dackman

When Eric's Mom Fought Cancer, Judith Vigna

When Life Become Precious, Elise NeeDell Babcock

When the Woman You Love Has Breast Cancer, Larry Eiler

Will I Get Breast Cancer? Questions and Answers for Teenage Girls, Carole Vogel

Woman to Woman, Hester Hill Schnipper and Joan Feinberg Berns

Appendix VI

Internet Resources

Appendix VI

Internet Resources

The following Internet resources are not all-inclusive. Also, given the progressive nature of the Internet, a particular site's addresses, content, or even existence may change. We suggest that you use this listing as a starting point for developing your own customized Internet resource library.

About Breast Cancer Resources
breastcancer.about.com

Alamo Breast Cancer Foundation
www.alamobreastcancer.org

Alpha Cancer Information Resource
www.alphacancer.com

AMC Cancer Research Center
www.amc.org

American Academy of Family Physicians
www.aafp.org

American Cancer Society
www2.cancer.org

American College of Obstetricians and Gynecologists
www.acog.com

American College of Radiology
www.acr.org

American Medical Women's Association
www.amwa-doc.org

American Pain Foundation
www.painfoundation.org

American Self-Help Clearinghouse
www.mentalhelp.net/selfhclp

American Society of Clinical Oncology
www.asco.org

American Society of Plastic and Reconstructive Surgeons
www.plasticsurgery.org

A Question Of Genes: Inherited Risks
www.pbs.org/gene

Artemis: The Johns Hopkins Breast Center E-Zine
www.med.jhu.edu/breastcenter/artemis

Ask NOAH About Cancer
www.noah-health.org

Association of Cancer Online Resources
www.acor.org

Blood and Marrow Transplant Newsletter
www.bmtnews.org

Breast Cancer Answers Project
www.canceranswers.org

Breast Cancer Center
www.patientcenters.com/breastcancer

Breast Cancer Lighthouse
www.commtechlab.msu.edu/sites/bcl

BreastCancer.Net
www.breastcancer.net

Breast Cancer Research
breast-cancer-research.com

Breast Cancer Resource Locator
www.thirdage.com/features/healthy/resource

Breast Cancer Risk Calculator
www.halls.md/breast/risk.htm

Breast Cancer Society of Canada
www.bcsc.ca

Breast Cancer Strategies
www.breastcancerstrategies.com

Breast Cancer Support Groups: CancerNews
www.cancernews.com/bcs.htm

Breast Cancer Survivors' Club
www.azstarnet.com/~pud/book/revised.html

Breast Cancer Voices From The Heart
healthtalk.com/bcen/voices.html

Cancer Care
www.cancercare.org

CancerEducation.com
www.cancereducation.com

Cancer News
www.cancernews.com

Cancer Guide: Steve Dunn's Cancer Information Page
www.cancerguide.org

Cancer Hope Network
www.cancerhopenetwork.org

CancerNet
www.cancernet.nci.nih.gov

CancerNews: Breast Cancer
www.cancernews.com/breast.htm

Cancerpage.com
www.cancerpage.com

Cancer Research Foundation of America
www.preventcancer.org

Centers for Disease Control and Prevention
www.cdc.gov/cancer/nbccedp

CenterWatch Clinical Trials Listing Service
www.centerwatch.com

Choice In Dying
www.choices.org

Cure Breast Cancer, Inc.
www.curebreastcancer.org

Department of Defense Breast Cancer Decision Guide
www.bcdg.org

Department of Health and Human Services Breast Cancer Area
www.os.dhhs.gov

Doctor's Guide to Breast Cancer Information
www.pslgroup.com/breastcancer.htm

Dr. Susan Love
www.susanlovemd.com

EduCare
www.cancerhelp.com

FORCE: Facing Our Risk of Cancer Empowered
www.facingourrisk.org

Health Talk Interactive
www.healthtalk.com

Health World Online
www.healthy.net

Inflammatory Breast Cancer Help Page
www.bestiary.com/ibc

Imaginis.com
www.imaginis.com

Intercultural Cancer Council
icc.bcm.tmc.edu

Leading Ladies
www.leadingladies.com

Lee National Denim Day
www.denimday.com

Living Beyond Breast Cancer
www.lbbc.org

Mautner Project
www.mautnerproject.org

MCW Healthlink: Breast Cancer
healthlink.mcw.edu/breast-cancer

Mid-Atlantic Breast Cancer Information Exchange
www.mabcie.com

National Alliance of Breast Cancer Organizations
www.nabco.org

National Asian Women's Health Organization
www.nawho.org

National Breast Cancer Awareness Month
www.nbcam.org

National Breast Cancer Coalition
www.natlbcc.org

National Cancer Institute
www.nci.nih.gov

National Center for Complementary and Alternative Medicine
www.nccam.nih.gov

National Coalition for Cancer Survivorship
www.cansearch.org

National Family Caregivers
www.nfcacares.org

National Institutes of Health Breast Cancer Patient Information
www.cancernet.nci.nih.gov/index.html

National Library of Medicine
www.nlm.nih.gov

National Lymphedema Network
www.lymphnet.org

National Self-Help Clearinghouse
www.selfhelpweb.org

National Women's Health Information Center
www.4women.gov

National Women's Health Resource Center
www.healthywomen.org

Native American Circle
www.mayo.edu/nativecircle

Nifty Fifty Breast Cancer Quilt
geocities.com/trequilts/charity.html

OncoChat: Online Support for Cancer Survivors, Families & Friends
www.oncochat.org

OncoLink – University of Pennsylvania Cancer Center
www.oncolink.upenn.edu

Oncology Nursing Society
www.ons.org

Patient Advocacy Groups Home Page
infonet.welch.jhu.edu/advocacy.html

SHARE, Self-Help for Women with Breast or Ovarian Cancer
www.sharecancersupport.org

thehealthchannel.com
www.thehealthchannel.com

The Libby Ross Foundation for Breast Cancer
www.thelibbyrossfoundation.com

The Susan G. Komen Breast Cancer Foundation
www.komen.org

The Wellness Community
www.wellnesscolumbus.org

Vital Options
www.vitaloptions.org

WebMedLit - Oncology
www.webmedlit.com

WellnessWeb Cancer Center
www.wellweb.com

Facts About Breast Cancer
www.cancerlinksusa.com/breast/wynk/index.htm

WIN Against Breast Cancer
winabc.org

Yahoo Alternative Medicine Index
www.yahoo.com/health/alternative_medicine

Y-ME
www.y-me.org

Young Survival Coalition
www.youngsurvival.org

My Notes

"My Favorite Internet Sites"
(And some important e-mail addresses too!)

_____

_____

_____

_____

_____

_____

_____

_____

_____

_____

_____

_____

Appendix VII

National Organizations

Appendix VII

National Organizations

AMC Cancer Research Center Cancer Information/ Counseling Line
1-800-525-3777

American Cancer Society
1-800-227-2345

American College of Radiology - Mammography Accreditation
1-800-227-6440

American Institute for Cancer Research
1-800-843-8114

American Society of Plastic and Reconstructive Surgeons
800-635-0635

American Society for Clinical Hypnosis
630-980-4740

Cancer Care
1-800-813-HOPE (4673)

Cancer Information Service (CIS) of the National Cancer Institute
1-800-4-CANCER

Food and Drug Administration, Breast Implant Information Line
1-888-463-6332

Lymphedema Network
1-800-541-3259

National Alliance of Breast Cancer Organizations
1-800-719-9154

National Breast Cancer Coalition
202-296-7477

National Coalition for Cancer Survivorship
1-877-622-7937

National Hospice Organization
1-800-658-8898

National Institutes of Health Library
301-496-2447

National Society of Genetic Counselors
610-872-7608

Office of Alternative Medicine, National Institutes of Health
1-888-644-6226

Share
212-719-0364

Sharing and Caring
1-888-649-9707

The Susan G. Komen Breast Cancer Foundation
1-800-I'M-AWARE (462-9273)

Y-ME
1-800-221-2141

My Notes

"Other Helpful Organizations"
(Including local groups and programs!)

_____

_____

_____

_____

_____

_____

_____

_____

_____

_____

_____

_____

INDEX

Index

A

B

C

S

T

U

V

Additional Order Form
for
"I Flunked My Mammogram!"

Would you like another copy of *"I Flunked My Mammogram!"* to send to a friend or loved one? Simply mail back the form below!

Name: _____

Address: _____

_____

_____

Quantity: _____ @ $11.95   per book

                    +   <u>$2.95</u> shipping & handling

                    = $14.90   per book (Maryland residents add 5%.)

Total Order: _____ x $14.90 = $ _____ .

Please make your check payable to
"I Flunked My Mammogram!"
and mail to:
"I Flunked My Mammogram!"
Post Office Box 307
Severna Park, Maryland 21146 USA

You can also order online by visiting
http://www.curebreastcancer.org
or call 1-888-371-1800